SILENT KILLERS

A Journey through the Complex Disorders
of Lyme Disease, Mold Toxicity,
Mercury Poisoning and Coronavirus

JENNIFER C. BROWER

Cover design: The concept for the book's cover was derived from evolving science, which will continue to improve our understanding of how our DNA, genetics and environment play into our overall health. The entire book team - author, editor, marketing manager and Nurse Practitioner - brainstormed together about a way to relay the whole story in an image. The body is made of so many things: genes and DNA and chromosomes which make us our unique selves.

FIRST EDITION
Printed in the United States of America

In Memory:

In loving memory of my parents, Martha Maguire Jennings and S. Bryan Jennings, Jr., and my sister Rebecca Pantelis. If I'd known then what I know now, none of them would have suffered from their illnesses to the degree they did.

Dedication:

To my children, Jennings, Darby, Jr. and Kendall, I would go to the ends of the earth for you, and you all taught me that I could also do that for myself. Leading from a place of strength as your Momma Bear, nothing was more important than protecting my cubs. Your love taught me that I needed to protect myself also.

To my husband, Darby, moving beyond fear, denial and repression takes incredible courage. In our 35 years of marriage, like all married couples, we have had times that we didn't like each other. But our love is so deep that we've dug to the core to find the grit needed to stick together through it all. We have beaten extraordinary odds, and I feel that God has a purpose for our lives together. I believe in my heart of hearts that I wrote this book for you, along with people everywhere to be encouraged to face hardships head-on, and move forward with the courage, strength and determination to be proactive in this gift of life as it unfolds before us. To this day, the tenets of our vows are "in sickness and in health," but I prefer that we strive for love, unity and wellness. I love you now, always and forever.

Table of Contents

Introduction

While this book is primarily about my health journey through Lyme and other infections, health challenges are not the only aspects of my life. In addition to being a wife, mother and avid exerciser, I was actually a rather successful businesswoman. A byproduct of my decades-long career in commercial real estate, which involved grand openings, was the opportunity to foray into the sports marketing events business. One day I was talking to friends who worked for the PGA tour and they shared that some ESPN scouts came to Jacksonville, Florida to find a location to host their Super Bowl XXXIX party. They were so disappointed by the lack of event venues that they planned to bus their guests from Disney World in Orlando to Jacksonville for the event! I knew there was a better solution. I contacted the scout and through an intricate negotiation, helped secure an amazing location directly next to the football stadium - St. Andrew's Episcopal Church, a small historical event center which also had a small park and a 100-year-old house. ESPN was able to completely renovate the house back to its original architecture and ultimately had a better venue than they'd ever imagined. We worked with every division of ESPN, including Magazine, TV, Sports and Entertainment, and we had the privilege of announcing ESPNU and introducing Alicia Keys to big-time fame. The project was a multi-day event which took months of hard work and planning, but everyone was very happy about how the event went. I tell this not to boast, but to emphasize that being sick and in a desperate search for wellness is not all there is to my story. Sadly, sickness and healing efforts can become the main storyline, as it did for me.

INTRODUCTION

In the darkest times of my illness and struggles, my faith in God buoyed me and helped me move forward. My hope is that this book will inspire you to achieve success in discovering where you find your healing. There may be times that you feel no one understands your pain as your body starts to fail. At times the fear you feel will be overwhelming and indescribable, as your soul is under attack. Find ways to allow peace to enter your life, be it through spiritual inspiration, encouragement, support groups, or any form of positive therapy that paves ways leading to resolve and healing.

Everyone has a story to share, and no one should ever be excluded from letting their voice be heard. Silence can be golden; indeed, I have been silent for many years. However, I know that now the time is right to tell my story. I once heard on a Ted Talk that "courage is fear walking." This resonated with me in such a way that I decided I would never allow fear and doubt to hold me back from sharing my experiences. Taking a silent approach is no longer an option for me. Too many people hurt in a similar way.

It is important that I share my journey with people who are living silently in fear and pain. Health struggles can seem confusing when you do not know where to turn. Whether you have obstacles relating to Lyme disease, cancer, or other diagnoses, it's comforting when you can relate to someone who's been pressured from many sides of a health crisis. I desire to help relieve the heaviness that's weighing on many hearts and point them in a supportive direction. If just by reading my story, only one person is saved from their current situation, my job is complete. If my story helps many, even better.

Simply put, I am here to help.

First and foremost, as soon as you recognize something "is off" in your body, and you can't remedy it, pay attention to your symptoms. When you initially notice there's a recurring, nagging problem, or the situation starts to affect you in your normal routines, take a few moments to assess yourself and find out what is really going on. Even though it may all be new to you at the moment, take a deep breath, and start writing down things that seem abnormal.

My symptoms were erratic - dizziness, headaches, trouble concentrating, and panic attacks. I began to feel burning in my brain. It was as if there were little bugs crawling around inside as I was trying to go to sleep. I begged my husband to help me because I was scared to death. It was like a constant movement yet an uncontrollable sensation. I could not even communicate correctly. Remember, the internet in 2007 was not what it is today for conducting research. I had to explain my symptoms over the phone to doctors. My fear was so great that I practically stopped eating because I didn't know what I could safely eat. All I knew to do was to research the little food that I was consuming on a daily basis. I talked to a nutritionist to learn if I was deficient in any areas and to address them accordingly. These steps helped me to get started on my healing journey before I even received any diagnosis. I was placed on an anti-inflammatory diet, and I was taken off dairy completely. I began juicing every day which included: ginger root, celery, cucumber, apple, carrot, cilantro, and a dark leafy green vegetable (kale or spinach). Movement was also recommended.

My primary care physician was a functional medical doctor, and she decided that in order to boost my immune system, she would start administering vitamins intravenously. It was fortunate that my doctor knew me when my health was best, even though I wasn't her patient at the time.

I was so freaked out when my symptoms came that it was hard to write many things down. I should have journaled my diet, exercise, thoughts, routines, and daily activities. In addition, it would have been great to include details of how to actively sort out difficult experiences and challenges that were altering my progress. I should have been logging daily and weekly goals, appointments, symptoms, clippings of research articles, what books I was reading, sleep patterns, disturbances during the night, medications (ones that had adverse effects *and* ones that worked), and resources that I could get connected to and had employed. It would be a personal health diary, and how useful it would have been! I did find it helpful as time passed to review doctors' notes to see how much progress I was making or if there were any setbacks. When you are encountering challenges with your health, take a quick moment to write it all out, if you can. It took me far too long to begin that critical practice. Please learn from my mistakes and force yourself to record every detail you possibly can from the beginning. Or at least get started now.

Looking back at all my experiences, sharing these pertinent moments in my journey, and offering you advice on potential treatments, my hope is to provide you with relief and positive results. As I share my story, my wish is that you recognize and accept that what works for one person may not work for another. Throughout my journey, I experienced many moments when others around me appeared to be healing at a faster rate. That was discouraging, causing negative thoughts to creep into my subconscious, and I had to pull myself back into positive healing thoughts to protect myself against personal pessimistic energies.

I encourage you to set your focus on your own individual healing and not worry about other people's progress. It is not a competition. It is *your* unique journey. Becoming engaged in how someone else heals and adapts to their treatment can cause you to lose sight of your own accomplishments. You can learn from others' experiences, but yours are unique and personal. To anyone who has been affected by Lyme disease, co-infections, mold toxicity, mercury poisoning and coronavirus, understand that these are complex disorders that medical professionals find tricky to resolve. And they don't affect only the person with the disease. Their tentacles extend way beyond the infected person and infiltrate every aspect of life in the most insidious manner. I hope that sharing my story will help you get to your journey's end as quickly, efficiently, and effectively as possible.

Brian Clement, Director of Hippocrates Wellness, provides expert commentary throughout this book. Please note that the positions he takes on various topics are his own.

Jennifer, like millions worldwide, is the victim of a new generation of diseases that in part stem from lifestyle habits and environmental concerns.

When she speaks of Lyme disease, this tick and insect-born disorder is only new on the scene and named after Lyme, Connecticut where it was first discovered in the mid-twentieth century. Bacterium Borrelia Burgdorferi is the medical name. There are also other species of Borrelia that cause this crippling disease.

When Jennifer addresses COVID-19 (SARS-Cov-2), she is speaking of a virus that has been created in a lab having several patents granted since the year 2000. The worldwide outbreak was first reported in December 2019 in the town of Wuhan Hubei Province, China, where the Chinese biowarfare laboratory has been in operation for more than eighty years and has conducted experiments with the U.S. government as well as other nations.

Mold disorders are a form of fungus whereas some varieties are producing mycotoxins which do not affect all people equally. Genetics testing reveals that there is a gene, which when absent, could cause severe health concerns.

Mercury toxicity is a serious heavy metal poisoning stemming from fish consumption, dental fillings, vaccines and many consumer products.

How this gathering of modern health destroyers is related is that each engages your immune system, and, like dominoes, collapses the whole anatomical system. Allopathic Physicians (MDs) are not educated in these new disorders and you must search for a provider who has become a specialist, often due to his or her own battle.

Brian Clement, PhD, LN.

Part 1: My Journey

Chapter 1

Darkness Strikes

By the beginning of 2020, back-to-normal life was returning to me. What relief I felt! Oh, the joy of getting energy back! But one day in February of 2020, the room went dark, my head was spinning, the aches were unbearable, and I just had to get my feet on the ground. NO, NO, NO! What was going on? Not again! Panic mode set in - I desperately needed 911. Could anyone hear me? Was this Lyme disease all over again? Please, no!

Whatever it was, this wave of illness put me right back in a place of fear. I could not get out of bed. The fear that had escaped me for years had returned. When I tried to stand up, the whole room spun, my head pounded, I couldn't take a deep breath, and I had to hold on to the walls to walk.

This was the beginning of another round of mysterious illness that would knock me down to the ground.

I was diagnosed with bronchitis, sinusitis, walking pneumonia, and throat infections. Doctors placed me on seven days of prednisone and strong antibiotics. They emphasized the importance of remaining stationary. I had no balance to begin with, so until the meds kicked in, I was trapped in my bed, except to get up to go to the bathroom. I panicked inside at the thoughts of Lyme disease attacking me again, but was something else triggering the disease that was possibly lying dormant? I'm here to share how COVID-19 revealed itself in my health and reactivated Lyme disease.

Welcome to the first round of cases of COVID-19. Recuperation took months. Regaining energy was a long struggle. I was juicing constantly and doing everything in my power to support my immune system. By summer I finally got back to exercising: doing reformer pilates and walking four to five miles a day. I was back to a semi-normal life, able to work again, and then two years later, *it attacked me a second time!* By the fall of 2022, the COVID-19 variant was different, and again my body felt broken into pieces. I had to attack it from a different angle so this infection would not stay with me like it did the first time. The burning in my feet was unbearable. Joint aches and brain fog, along with the co-infections of Lyme, were symptoms I had not experienced for years in my battles, but they were reignited. Some of the symptoms such as joint aches were more excruciating with the second battle of COVID-19.

> COVID-19 is an RNA virus and alters unfamiliar areas of your immunity, therefore disturbing your natural fighter and killer cells that work in concord with the T-cells (general). This is a collaboration that is required to hold Lyme symptoms at bay.
>
> Brian Clement, PhD, LN.

Since I was not able to sustain my health after the two COVID battles, I searched for a wellness center that could treat me holistically, considering all I'd learned from previous, collective treatments. I wanted all the healing under one roof. I had studied Hippocrates Wellness in West Palm Beach, Florida for years. Then, honestly, I forgot about it.

My 2022 bout with COVID-19 triggered an aha! moment as I remembered that Hippocrates Wellness offered all the things I needed: nutrition, IV, lifestyle changes, doctors and treatment in one place at the same time. My first visit was in December of 2022. I thought I was going into the 21-day life transformation program, but I went into the immunity protocol program instead. I was invited to a meeting led by Brian Clement, PhD, LN., on causes of cancer and its effect on the immune system. I began working on recovering and developing more tools to increase my immune system. I began my post-COVID protocol that was 2 months long after my second visit to Hippocrates Wellness. I was going to beat this hell in a different way this time. There were so many people dying from COVID and Lyme disease, and I refused to be added to the list of innocent, vulnerable lives lost due to affliction with these deadly bugs and viruses.

In this world, we constantly face battles. Our mind, our physical body and perhaps even our spirit encounter and endure many tribulations. Illness seems to pose greater challenges for some than for others. There are many stories and situations that have lasted longer due to COVID-19, and the effects in some cases have been devastating. Whether vaccinated or not, whether you've had COVID-19 once, multiple times, or not at all, we all may share some of the same feelings.

Have you ever thought about the moment you realized that something wasn't right? You could not put your thoughts together. It was too difficult to explain. You sounded like a crazy person, and others developed erroneous perceptions about you. I know exactly how that feels.

This is what darkness looks like when it strikes: the problems lie before you and you have no answers. A deep sense of confusion and worry, constant turmoil, and the weight of the world seems to sit on your shoulders.

I felt that I was living in a flume of dust and confusion. The fact is that COVID-19 reactivated the fears of Lyme and mold.

> Conventional physicians can often face illnesses that they are not familiar with and react by labeling them "mental disorders." Inherently this spills over to your family and friends who at times detach and concur with the doctor.
>
> Brian Clement, PhD, LN.

Let's go back to the year 2010. It began to sink in that something was happening inside of me. A painful sensation in my brain would interfere with making sense of the situation at hand. My brain felt as if it were being fried or plugged into an electrical outlet. The extreme pressure in my brain was as if a solid cloud were taking shape in thickness and form. Even in my quiet moments, thoughts were racing all around me causing panic and increasing anxiety. Have you ever had a pain somewhere in your body and you were unable to pinpoint the actual location? That is how I felt many times! When a baby shrieks in a high-pitched audible sound, he is verbalizing his discomfort the only way he can. There are many times that I felt like shrieking, but it often came out in tears of frustration and fear.

A neighbor came by one day to bring me an article about the dangers of mercury amalgams (fillings) in your teeth. The article stated that they could affect your autoimmune system and weaken your fighting mechanisms.

I recently read on Healthline.com that "Mercury is a type of toxic metal that we can come into contact with in a variety of ways. This may include consuming certain types of seafood and wearing certain types of jewelry. The most common cause of mercury poisoning is from consuming too much methylmercury or organic mercury, which is linked to eating seafood. Mercury itself is naturally occurring, but the amounts in the environment have been on the rise due to industrialization. The metal can make its way into soil and water, and eventually into animals like fish. Consuming foods with mercury is a common cause of this type of poisoning."

I was not interested in having anything inside my mouth made from mercury! I made an appointment with my dentist to discuss having my seven fillings removed and replaced with composite. Though he said that he was very aware of the precautions to take, he did not. I was left with tremendous pain after having the fillings removed incorrectly. The intensity I felt was like having ice picks stabbed into my brain, specifically my frontal lobe. We called the dentist back to ask why I was having this feeling. He said that he possibly hit a nerve with the Novocain, but what really happened was there was no "boot" in my mouth or full oxygen mask over my nose during the procedure. I ingested mercury gasses into my nasal passages, and mercury lodged into my frontal lobe. Tests confirmed years later that my mercury levels were elevated.

I met a holistic dentist at Hippocrates Wellness who was speaking on the correct way to safely remove mercury amalgams. Her name is Dr. Marianna Kaufman, and I asked her to summarize her position and protocol.

Dr. Marianna Kaufman

It has been well established that, of all the non-radioactive elements on this planet, mercury is the most toxic. It is a strong neurotoxin and burdens the immune system. So why do so many dentists across the world still place fillings containing this poisonous substance? In fact, mercury was first introduced as a useful addition to metallic fillings in the early 1800's. Its benefits included low cost and ease of use.

Mercury is a liquid metal, and as such, it provided a pliability to the filling material which made for improved handling properties. At a time that gold was the only alternative, mercury/silver fillings became an affordable solution for the masses. Today, we have far more options available to us. Resins and ceramics can certainly be deemed the standards of care in today's dental practices, but why do mercury fillings still subsist? The European Parliament has voted to ban mercury-containing fillings, with the total ban taking effect in 2025. Thus far, however, the United States has made no indication of a similar such move. The official stance of the ADA (American Dental Association) and the FDA is that mercury-containing fillings offer the same safety class as resin and gold. Although, the FDA does mention that the vapor released from these fillings may lead to inhalation and potential lung damage if the levels are high enough.

As a Holistic and Physiological Dentist, I am a member of a minority of dentists who do not subscribe to the safety of amalgams. I consider the term "silver filling" to be an overt misnomer given the fact that these fillings are 50%+ mercury and only 35% silver. And while I am not in a position to persuade our legislators, I do consider it my duty to educate people on the critical importance of safety during removal of these restorations. As has been conceded by the FDA, inhalation of mercury is considered to be the most harmful method of exposure. The question of how much mercury vapor is emitted when eating on these fillings or by brushing them with a toothbrush has not been established; however, we do know that the removal of these mercury-containing fillings generates a high amount of vaporization (emission of small particles which can be easily inhaled).

This is where I step in. No restoration is designed to last forever. The mouth is a high wear-and-tear environment and dentistry should be viewed as a temporary solution. Whether a tooth has a failing mercury filling which requires replacement or if my patient is seeking elective removal, I believe a strict safety protocol is crucial. Remember: Inhalation is the most harmful method of exposure! When we talk about the removal of mercury fillings what we are really saying is that they will be drilled out. Our dental drill is essentially a tool of vaporization. This cannot be stated emphatically enough!

In my opinion, protection against inhalation during the removal of mercury fillings should be the standard of care. It is not. In my practice I employ the S.M.A.R.T. (Safe Mercury Amalgam Removal Technique) protocol established by the IAOMT (International Academy of Oral Medicine and Toxicology). This approach is designed to protect both the patient and the dental team from mercury exposure during removal. When patients seek me out for their mercury filling removal treatment, this is what they can expect:

- Oxygen mask with direct pressure flow

- Isolation of the tooth or teeth which contain mercury by using a dental dam. This dam should block out the rest of the entire oral cavity. No adjacent teeth, gums, tongue or throat can be seen

- Impermeable barriers are placed over the entire patient body including all skin, clothing, and hair and are tucked under the dental dam

- An extra-oral vacuum (large diameter strong vacuum tube) with HEPA and Charcoal filtration is placed as close as possible to the patient's mouth during removal

- Sectioning of the mercury filling into large chunks to minimize drilling amount and subsequent vaporization

- Decontamination of all instruments and equipment before continuing to the next step of dental visit

In addition to these safety measures, my assistant and I wear positive pressure hoods during these procedures. This is much of what I do. I take my position very seriously and am always eager to educate people on this topic, both in my practice and during my lectures. We know that the mouth is often a window through which we can assess the health of the entire body. In addition to its close proximity to the throat, sinuses, and brain, the tissues of the mouth are highly vascular (a lot of blood vessels), which leads to quick and deep absorption. A healthy body cannot be established without a healthy mouth.

Mercury is second only to radiation as a poisonous disease-causing element. By eating away at the nerves and destroying immune system cells, it plays havoc with your overall health.

Brian Clement, PhD, LN.

The fiery sensation inside my brain was something I didn't understand. The pain in my joints, feet, and the inability to concentrate left me begging for help from my husband, father, and mother-in-law. There was a tortured feeling within me pleading for relief. *My body was malfunctioning.* It felt like I was screaming inside and out, but I wasn't able to get the sound out to explain what was occurring. My spinal cord was shaking, and I could not voice the absolute fear that I was experiencing. God help me! Why am I going through this? No sleep – no rest – no internal peace. It was hard to rationalize everything that was going on.

Most of my closest friends and family members did not understand why I could not handle or manage "it", whatever that "it" was. The disease itself, taking care of my kids, my husband, my responsibilities - it was challenging to manage "it." Honestly, I *wanted* to handle "it" too! Constantly questioning myself, life began to unravel. The fear in my mind was unnerving. Making sense of the confusion and pain was overwhelming. I was going down.

During this time, my extended family thought I was literally going crazy! To help, my sister Terry created a working calendar for me to stay organized with taking medications, my kids' schedules, and errands. I went months without sleeping. My head felt like it was gone! I was on so much medication, and taking notes during treatments was overwhelming. The book was created in order to have a well-detailed plan. All sorts of material were included that could be used in research, diet, and daily schedule. Terry stayed with me for weeks to help me get through life. She kept a list of all my medications, helped with my kids, and ensured everything was charted. Action statements were outlined in my book such as:

- focus on the day ahead

- think through your anxiety

- break the cycle

- set your goals the day before and write them down

- focus on your environment

- stay busy doing the things you love

Before the diagnosis of Lyme disease and the inflicting ailments of mold toxicity, I could never have imagined or prepared for life to be turned upside down. The gates of hell seemed to be opening all around me. Portals of negativity, conflict, pitfalls, blockages, and hindrances were against me constantly. Healing was on the other side, but it seemed impossibly far away.

We are designed to face the adversities of life that try to interfere with our natural and human process of living freely. An illness puts us to the test. It is then our job to fight and win the battle. When you feel like the wind has been knocked out of you, parts of the day feel like out-of-body experiences and you're caught in a web of infirmities, all you want to do is scream for help.

Being ill with Lyme was lonely and isolating, and I often felt unsupported and unloved. Loneliness, stress and fear were my constant companions. The disease infiltrated my mind, body and soul, and the illness became more controlling and dominating as time went by. Any prospect of a normal life was bleak at this point, and many people could not see or understand what I was experiencing internally and physically. It became a constant challenge of finding the hope and courage to push myself and remain optimistic that it wouldn't last forever. I would say to myself that this illness was not going to get the best of me; I would do whatever it took to beat it! I went through many trials and tribulations to move forward, but often gave up hope.

Not only had I lost far too much weight at this point, but the hopelessness I saw in my own eyes scared and angered me. I would think to myself, what other areas in my life are stifled because of the pain, and what will it take to unleash the sorrows and return to who I really am? I felt tremendous despair, but fortunately, I was still a determined woman. I knew this natural commitment to self would lead me in a new direction.

> Comprehensive interconnection of all of self is a clear science called psychoneuroimmunology. Systemic connection between your organs, immune cells and mind is understood and addressed by advanced practitioners.
>
> Brian Clement, PhD, LN.

It's tempting to place our hands over our ears and shut our eyes in an attempt to avoid confronting our painful health reality. But not only is that not sustainable, it's surrendering to defeat. We have to start within ourselves. I would generate vibrational energy by talking to myself and repeating positive mantras, such as, "I am a strong, healthy, and vibrant woman." Positive energies help affirm that you can make it through the toughest challenges. You may want to come up with your own affirmation to repeat every day to ensure that your body is receiving positive reinforcement from within.

> Mindfulness research discovered that affirmative techniques can increase activation and numbers of immune cells by as much as 40% in only five minutes.
>
> Brian Clement, PhD, LN.

In order to start moving forward, you need help formulating an action plan. Everyone's action plan is different based on individual needs. Keep your mind active with positive things, exercise daily, eat healthfully as much as possible, find support groups, and take deep breaths when you feel anxiety rise within you. Make daily goals that are attainable and write down your feelings. These small but impactful actions will help you along the way.

Chapter 2

Starting the Search

The body is such a unique entity that even to this day, scientists are continuously mesmerized by it. Our bodies are designed carefully and organized into many systems that are intended to function as they should. Everyone has his or her own genetic makeup. Cells, tissues, and organs are developed into an array of multifaceted instruments of an original masterpiece. The way we heal and recover can depend on our body structure and physical composition. Our body is alarmed when foreign substances try to take root and trigger negative imbalances. This is the place at which our bodies begin to struggle with healing, and intervention is needed.

I was physically and emotionally in turmoil. I saw many doctors in hopes that they could navigate and treat my symptoms as well as provide a diagnosis. Autoimmune specialists at the Mayo Clinic in Jacksonville ran numerous blood tests, and after a lumbar spinal tap, they concluded that I had meningitis and said to go home and rest. Other doctors at Mayo, as well as doctors at many well-respected medical institutions across the country, threw around a flurry of diagnostic theories: Rocky Mountain Spotted Fever, Epstein-Barr, viral meningitis, fibromyalgia, and depression. *All of which I found out later were co-infections of Lyme.*

Lyme is difficult to diagnose. Multiple doctors have told me that other diseases are significantly easier to diagnose and treat. Since Lyme does not follow the same course for everyone, it requires a very specific blood test and often other tests that do not meet the scope of insurance approvals. Additionally, I was told by many doctors that there is no way I could have Lyme disease because "it's not in Florida." Yet a research scientist that I met at the Northeast Florida Lyme council meeting informed me that about 200,000 cases existed in northeast Florida alone (Florida Times-Union, 2011). After consulting with him, we decided to gather blood samples and do urine tests, hoping to better understand what was happening to my body. Although the scientist could not explain the intense burning in my brain associated with my symptoms, it was obvious that there was great interference with my physical abilities. He did what he could for me. At this point, I still felt that I was getting nowhere.

An infectious disease specialist from the Columbia-Presbyterian Hospital in New York City told me I did not have enough symptoms to be diagnosed with Lyme disease; plus, *I was from Florida.* How many other doctors had misdiagnosed me?

Many stressful life events occurred simultaneously. My mother passed away at Christmastime in 2007 and on the same day of her death, I received a call regarding a concern over a recent mammogram. I had an emergency lumpectomy in my left breast just days before my mother's funeral. Even though I endured all of this pain, my real struggle was still very deep, dark, and lonely. It seemed like the doors of hell were swinging wide open. It is very common for people with autoimmune issues to experience flareups during extremely stressful life events.

On a trip to Maine in 2010, a group of trusted girlfriends shared that they were convinced I had Lyme disease. They pinpointed the neurological sensitivity I had as something they knew others with the Lyme diagnosis had experienced. After I returned home, I went for testing and my results lit up like a Christmas tree. Eureka! After years of going to the doctors, I finally had a diagnosis! My personal theory is that I contracted Lyme through a spider bite in 1998. At the time I was in southwest Florida on my tenth wedding anniversary trip, and I remember the bite. It is the only time I can recall not being able to get out of bed or move for multiple consecutive days.

Some areas of my life were so peculiar and misunderstood that they caused me to put up walls that would be hard for anyone to break down. These walls were erected as safety nets so no one could see the real pain I was in. Others may use their walls as defense due to past hurt or trauma when trust was destroyed. Some may do it because that's all they know. We keep life's struggles so hidden that once we do share them, people have a hard time believing us. Sometimes we can be so numb to our own pain that we forget how long we've been carrying it. Embarrassment, humiliation, shame, guilt, or just plain fear can prevent us from opening up. We're afraid of being judged.

We tend to forget what we have overcome in life. The very thing that could destroy our homes, families or relationships can actually bring strength, courage, and freedom. Someone else may be going through the same thing and having a rough time finding comfort. I often felt that I was going crazy, and I wanted my husband, Darby, to help me. His most common response was that he had to go to the office and get to work. It's true that his income was helping to fund my myriad treatments, but it still hurt that he would just leave me standing there, shattered. It seemed that neither he nor anyone else understood how I was feeling or what I was going through. I felt angry that there was no contribution from him in finding a solution for my healing. Fear prevented Darby from accepting that his wife was very ill and different from the woman he married, and frankly, he was running from it instead of dealing with it.

No one could see us sinking. Neither my husband nor I understood how we nearly allowed each other to drown in our own deep ends of fear. Nothing could heal our hearts at this moment. I didn't know if things would ever get back to normal or if I would ever be the real me or see my husband the same way. We both felt lost.

I believe that God uses our past stories to help others and bring freedom to their lives. We've all gone through things that are not easy to share with people. This long, painful season of my life caused me to fall to my knees every day. I didn't know where my saving help was going to come from. My life was a total nightmare.

When someone has a disease that attacks their autoimmune system, it's natural to be afraid of all sorts of things in their environment. The street that we lived on had exposed power lines, and the transformer was only 50 feet from our bedroom. I could hear the buzzing and feel the sensation of electricity. My father and sisters suggested that I move in with my sister who lived a mile away. I lived with Bonnie for a few weeks trying to heal and get myself back together. But it was difficult to live apart from my children and Darby, so I moved back home. We met with the powerline company to discuss the transformer, and with neighborhood support we were able to get the power lines put underground approximately a year later.

> Electropollution is a well-researched and established fact that impacts our overall health. Close proximity to electric plants, high tension wires, 5G and even wall sockets weaken one's endurance, adding to the potential of increased symptoms and disease.
>
> Brian Clement, PhD, LN.

Through all of this, I continued to pursue treatment for Lyme. However, I was not getting any better. One day my daughter Kendall decided to play dress up and went into a bedroom closet to find my dresses. When she pulled them back, we found that the closet wall was covered in black mold! We didn't know the dangers of living in a house with mold. The mold toxicity had physical effects on all five of my family members that I was unaware of at the time.

I was so self-consumed with the struggles of being sick that I did not see the stress and pressure my husband was under, or what was mounting with his career. Thinking their joint business was highly valued and that the market was ripe, Darby's business partner became hell-bent on selling the business. He started to pressure Darby to the point that my husband was experiencing sleepless nights and extreme anxiety. He ended up hospitalized for a couple weeks, which for me felt like an eternity. The reality of the anguish that he was dealing with shocked me and left me feeling helpless, hurt, and alone. In fact, I *was* alone. Home alone, very ill and with three children who did not know where Dad had gone. I lied to our children and everyone else, saying that their father had been in a car accident and that he would soon be released from the hospital. I felt that he should be the one to share with our children what truly happened once he felt grounded enough to do so.

Once he returned home, we sat our children down for a serious conversation, and Darby explained why he'd been gone so long. What an eye-opener their reaction was to us both. They were relieved! All that time my kids were afraid we were getting a divorce. We were surprised by the impact on them of their friends' parents splitting up. As long as we were staying together, they could digest any other news.

Having to face so many crises made our family more thankful for each other and made us realize that we could overcome anything together. Our relationships were reinforced, and we became more supportive of one another. I am mindful that 90% of marriages that encounter such travesty fail, and I am grateful to be in the rare 10%.

Chapter 3

Transitioning Into the Unknown

Prior to my panic attacks, I felt extremely competent and capable of taking excellent care of not only myself but my family. I rarely relied on others for any sort of assistance in my personal or professional life. Working out, playing tennis and socially coordinating events for my children, husband, and career were regular routines in my life. Being a businesswoman parenting three children and married to a workaholic, my social calendar was always full. Stress was a constant factor, but my overall life was awesome and fulfilling.

Remember that in 2005 I traveled to the New York Sports Symposium? Well, there's more to that story. On the flight home, while we waited for clearance on the tarmac, seconds turned into hours in my mind. I felt as if I were closed in a coffin, with no air, and confined in space. I started unbuttoning my shirt and hyperventilating. I was having a real panic attack. My business partner and I were not seated together, and the woman next to me, who happened to have been a yoga instructor, realized what was happening and started to calm me down using breathing techniques. I had to close my eyes and change my focus, envisioning the ocean and imagining my body in the salt water. I started focusing on other passengers in the plane rather than myself. Eventually the panic subsided.

A few weeks later, my business partner and I were at a lunch meeting and everything on my right side (arm and leg) began going numb. I couldn't even get my mouth to work properly, as my speech seemed to be impaired. Thank God my partner knew me so well, she could see I was in distress. She used my phone and called 911. I was rushed to the emergency room at Mayo Clinic. They thought I had a stroke and began to run numerous blood tests.

My husband returned from a business conference in Ohio to find me in the ER. The doctors had done a lumbar spinal tap and determined that I had viral meningitis. The doctor, who was a resident, released me with no help, and after the fact, others and I felt that I should not have been released from the hospital. I went home with no medications and my health did not improve.

Today's number 3 killer is modern medicine. Between the general collapse of the public's immunity, the plethora of new disorders and a total lack of doctors keeping up with the latest science, we are all placed in an untenable situation.

Brian Clement, PhD, LN.

Later that night I experienced the strangest and scariest dream of my life. I was driving my car along a paved road in a neighborhood that eventually turned into a dirt road. All of the houses around me began to disappear. It seemed that the times of the day changed drastically, from light to dark. I was in total darkness. I could no longer see anything around me. All of a sudden, my car began to plunge into a deep, dark hole. It was as if I were no longer in control of my path to veer back or reverse my direction. I was trapped with no way to get out. The mud had closed me in on all sides. My efforts to remove myself from this tragic dream would not release me from the darkness that surrounded me. I felt like I was suffocating, and my life was coming to an end. I forced myself to wake up, but I still felt locked down physically, while I was trying to convince myself that I was awake. I began to ponder what it actually meant to dream so vividly about a situation that appeared to have the same effects on me in the physical and natural world. It was as if life were closing in on me and all attempts to escape from this gruesome pressure were keeping me bound and enclosed.

The nights were long and dreadful. My attempts at sleep coincided with lightning flashes of white and silver light behind my eyelids. I couldn't wait to see the sunrise. I was feeling extremely weak and unstable. I felt like my central nervous system was completely haywire. The nerves inside my brain must have been sending the wrong signals! The conditions I was experiencing started to get the best of me. I would lie on the floor in my bathroom holding my Bible and praying to God to relieve me of this sickness. I would question Him as to why I was being tortured with this hell.

Although I had many horrible days and sleepless nights, I just pushed and pushed. I was in constant turmoil and my psychological state was shredded. As my condition deteriorated, my children became worried about me. I saw the fear and confusion in their eyes. Looking back, I can articulate and understand that making it through these phases and experiences in my life were steps needed to move in the right direction. My staunch faith in God buoyed me through the physical and mental pain, and without it, I am not sure I would be here today. Even though I knew all of this, the pain was still inevitable, and it felt that it would not be easing up any time soon.

My husband was concerned about me, but as he is consistently practical, he often asked me why I could not just be treated locally. And of course, it made more sense to go with providers covered by our insurance. Yet there were very few treatment centers locally that could provide the services I needed. Even after years of effective treatments, my husband would constantly question why I had the need for more treatments. Getting better was my main focus at the time. The fact of the matter is that doctors and clinics that specialize in treating Lyme disease successfully (that is, *medically* successfully) often do not take insurance and expect payment at the time of treatment. This was building contention between the two of us. Darby was tired of hearing about the disease and was frustrated with my plateauing. His stress was not just for what I was going through, but that he was unable to help or find the answers I needed.

Trying to get anyone else to understand what I was thinking or going through was a challenge all in itself. But I would pursue my journey with or without anyone's help. Being fed up with the condition of my health, I came to a crucial point. I was no longer seeking the opinions of others for my solution. It was time to take matters into my own hands.

Back in 2008, I found a healing center in Thomasson, Georgia called Be in Health that was strictly based on the principles of the Bible. This place opened so much spiritual insight into my life when I felt that I was at a breaking point. Not only was I spiritually dying, but it felt physical. The constant draining within me came with a strong desire to release hidden emotions that had much to do with my physical ailments. Though not everything was resolved after attending the healing conference, this time in my life was used as a reference to reflect on how far I had come and to look at the journey ahead.

My mother-in-law, Karen, was diagnosed with stage 4 lung cancer, and found a treatment center in Mesa, Arizona called An Oasis of Healing. Initially, I went with her to relieve my father-in-law for a month while he stayed at home. I was humbled to be of support to my mother-in-law throughout her healing journey.

While at the Oasis, I joined Karen on the green juice fast, which was a part of her treatment. I also began to build my own relationships with the doctors and staff. It became apparent to them that I was battling in my body as well. The doctors put their heads together and started treating me too. I enthusiastically accepted the opportunity for an experience of wellness. This was the beginning of new hope.

With a treatment plan developed, I began IV therapy to treat my immune system with magnesium. This was a great source of pain relief. Other treatment methods I underwent were colonic therapy, myofascial release, acupuncture, lymphatic drainage, the use of infrared sauna and ozone machine, foot bath treatments, and nutritional guidance. In efforts to try for ultimate relief and healing, this was the full onset of entering the world of non-traditional medicine. Even during this time, I felt that the ozone therapy was helpful in eliminating a lot of my pain and provided more clarity in my thought process. It was such a unique therapy that it was generally found only in holistic practices. Then there became a point at which I could feel my body responding to what I was receiving.

I took advantage of the morning walks to the clinic, as the place we rented was about a mile away. Walking prepared me for the day's journey of being plugged up to IV's all day and setting the tone of meeting the new patients coming in. We were all placed in the same room and had no choice but to stare at each other all day. No electronic devices were allowed. Making social connections was something

I was really great at doing. Taking advantage of each moment I had with others brought inner joy for me. The staff sat me near the grumpiest patients in the room, and I'm pretty sure that was on purpose. I never took for granted whom I sat by, as these moments were used to teach us all something.

At times I felt my place was to help those angrier patients change their mindsets for the better. We know that when people are not well, they tend to have doubts about their healing. At one point I joked that the staff should pay me to boost up the patients. One day, a really over-confident patient was on his computer during treatment, refusing to abide by the no-technology rules. Then he got the call to go to his colonic session. When he returned to the room, somehow it was so funny to everyone that we knew exactly where he had just come from. The whole room was laughing, including the doctors and staff, and eventually Mr. Confident himself. We needed this moment! This is what a normal day was like at Oasis.

I was always the last patient to receive my bags of treatment. The nurses would find the time to sit with me and would enjoy conversations at the end of the day. The point of being there was to heal and lift others up while we were all healing. The support of one another was vital in this clinic. We were each other's support through the constant change of patients checking in and out of the center. This initial journey set me up to see what was lying ahead. I admit that it was scary, and the unknown was baffling. Initially, I was there for a total of four weeks.

> Our perception of need leads us to believe that an endless search to receive is required. Ironically, the opposite works whereas when you freely express passionately, your heart opens and healing love increases.
>
> Brian Clement, PhD, LN.

Six months later I returned to the clinic along with my friend who was dangerously suicidal. We started on the green juice diet (my second round of the diet) and lost a lot of weight. I never realized that I shouldn't have been walking so much while on the green juice diet until my pants started falling off of me! Nevertheless, going through different protocols to find out what would work best for me, we concluded that higher doses of magnesium relieved most of my pain. The two doctors at An Oasis of Healing made a major difference in my life.

Another interesting fact about this unique place was that all of the food came directly from the center. The patients would take home the food made for them on a daily basis. The green juice I was given came in a three-quart bottle that was so thick it was challenging to get it all down, but I managed. Seeing the benefits and manifestation of what the foods and drinks did enabled my inner healing process to speed up. This is why it is so important to have a great diet while undergoing treatment of any kind.

I would also like to highlight a special type of treatment that was performed on patients at the Oasis. Insulated Potential Therapy (IPT) was done on patients who had cancer. They were given ice cold gloves to place on their hands and cold coverings for their head and feet. The heat of the body mixed with the cold would initiate a healing mechanism. Their internal temperature was lowered as if in a diabetic state. After that, they were given a cookie, followed by a low dose of chemotherapy, which would go to the cancer site. The cancer cells would open because of the sugar in the cookie. While in the diabetic state, and as the body was warming back up, the sugar components in the cookie would bind to the cancer cells. In efforts to attack the cancer cells, the blood in the body would begin to repair. Along with low doses of chemotherapy, IV minerals would be given to help remove those dead particles from the cells that were attacked. This was quite an interesting technique that was used to warm and cool the body in efforts to restore and heal from difficult diseases, such as cancer.

> Unlike healthy normal cells, cancer has eighty times more receptors for sugar, leading science to acknowledge that all forms are the fuel that provokes cancer's growth (metastasize).
>
> Brian Clement, PhD, LN.

The Neurological Institute of Columbia University diagnosed me with aseptic meningitis of presumed viral origin, chronic post-meningitis, daily headaches (migraine type), and history of positive Lyme serology. At this point, I had received so many different diagnoses over a short period of time, that I began to question the scopes of practicing physicians. Not only was this whole journey crazy in this aspect, but it was extremely consuming to go through countless physicians and be told one thing after another. This may seem pretty basic, but a difference exists between doctors and scientists, as well as medicine and science.

The other thing that intrigues me to this day is how many of these physicians are no longer in business. They all provided me with some form of treatment and aided in my journey. A majority of the physicians did what they knew to do. Looking back now I can definitely say that nothing was done in vain. I went through these treatment facilities for a reason.

There are many things I wish I knew then that I know now. I have gained so much wisdom and insight into the mechanisms of how treatments work. At times I wonder, would things be different for me now if I had just stayed the course and worked with my initial physician? While reflecting back on my healing journey, there was one particular doctor who did multiple protocols to build my immune system. Dr. Julie Buckley was an amazing and brilliant physician who operated with expertise and profound knowledge. Her specialty was elaborate in treating autism and other difficult diseases. She is a dear friend and the first doctor who was willing to try to discover whatever was happening in me. She even cured her own daughter from autism and herself from breast cancer! My appreciation goes out to her, and I recognize her ability to provide healing for people all over the world. Focusing on healing from Lyme disease had not surfaced fully in her practice; therefore, my treatments with her were limited at the time.

About three years later I received an unexpected call from a scientist at the University of North Florida who reached out to tell me that he had experienced the same symptoms that I had originally. To my surprise, while going through drastic changes, he revealed that he was at a crashing point in his own life. He regularly checked in with me to consult about my opinions regarding various treatments. I began investigating many options. It was at this moment that I considered pursuing science rather than medicine.

My first focus became to replenish my body. The benefits of healing myself started with a daily routine. Getting up early and fighting through the exhaustion that plagued my body, it was vital for me to recover from the sleepless nights. Taking vitamins, supplements, and staying hydrated were key to revitalizing my cells. IV drips were a big deal for me. I wanted to ensure that my mornings began early with a nice two-mile walk around the neighborhood. I flooded my body with freshly squeezed celery juice. Reading books was a great way to wind down after the busyness of my afternoon appointments.

> When ill, it is imperative that we remain rested, nourished, calm and mobile.
>
> Brian Clement, PhD, LN.

Taking control of what I knew to do was the best way I could stay afloat and balance daily routines. I didn't want anyone to see me crumble. Whatever I needed to do just had to be done, no matter how depleted or unenergized my body felt. Pushing through the throbbing headaches, body aches and imbalances, and all the fogginess in the brain, the key to my longevity was having an organized daily plan. Trust me, there were times that I just wanted to keep the blinds closed, pull the covers back over my head, turn the notifications off of my phone, cancel all my meetings, and not engage with anyone.

The constant draining sensation that flooded my body with all of the Lyme symptoms caused major interruptions throughout my day. There were times I just could not think clearly enough to get through major conversations or duties. I didn't always listen to my body or follow the signs. Especially as mothers and wives, we have to consistently be on the move. If we aren't, everything at home can fall to pieces. Thankfully, during these moments, I could take a break in my car, close my eyes, and just sit in the stillness. Tears would fall out of desperation for this journey to end, and the fight for healing would rest heavily on my shoulders.

Discerning appropriate treatment ended up being at least as hard, if not harder than getting the diagnosis. I worked with a Lyme specialist in my hometown, and she took me as far as she could. Her efforts brought me only some relief. Many times after that I would work with a doctor, plateau with their treatments, and then need to work with yet another doctor. All of their approaches to Lyme disease came from different angles.

It's ok to step out into the world of the unknown when it comes to getting better. Answers are not always at your fingertips, and researching takes a great deal of time and energy. I know what it feels like to keep searching because one answer is just not enough. Sometimes, the traditional methods simply don't work. What lies around the corner may be something no one around you has ever thought of or attempted to try.

Chapter 4

Electro-Sensitivity

Have you ever felt that you may have a sensitivity to Wi-Fi or certain electronic devices? Or have you experienced an odd sensation when around high electrical currents? I discovered some years ago that my body was overly sensitive to having Wi-Fi connected in my home. I started experiencing unexplainable headaches, lack of sleep, ringing in my head, extra fuzziness, and a sensitivity to sound reactions.

I am aware that this topic may be uncomfortable for people, especially those who have experienced similar issues. It is not widely discussed, but it is real. A man from church who knew some of my sensitivities approached me and timidly explained that he was concerned because of the onset of horrible headaches, and at times he experienced a brain-body disconnection, especially when in his car. Mid-drive he would forget how to get where he was going, even when it was a place he went to frequently. I told him he needs to pull over and get out of his car to ground himself by taking off his shoes and putting his bare feet on earth - grass, sand, dirt, etc. I explained to him that often this can be a reaction of the brain to the effects of bluetooth from the car. At one point in the past, I even had my car dealership do a rewiring of copper in my vehicle's dashboard to lower the Bluetooth connections. This helped reduce the frequency exposure to electromagnetic fields.

> Dr. Hardell, a Swedish oncologist and world-leading expert in the field of EMF radiation disease, has spearheaded the science community's research in the area of physical maladies connected to electronic pollution. Dr. Devra Davis is the lead scientist in the U.S. working with the University of Colorado, Stanford, Yale and others exposing the many disorders that these renegade frequencies cause.
>
> Brian Clement, PhD, LN.

When a person develops a sensitivity to electronic devices, they become sensitive to external and internal factors in their surrounding environments. The causes of reactions may vary depending on the nature of the stimulant. Our senses can help us detect what causes our bodies to become imbalanced. In terms of electro-sensitivity, it is an occurrence that relates to someone having a low tolerance towards energy fields such as Wi-Fi, Bluetooth, etc. The currents of electromagnetic fields may affect one's central nervous system and create a vibration or internal shaking that creates fight or flight mode. The frequency prevents the nervous system from calming down and can affect the sleep cycle. The experiences of strong electrical sensations, burning, and painful vibrations in my brain were unbearable. Yet, no one could tell me why I felt it or give a reasonable answer.

I am so electro-sensitive that I can walk into any home or building and locate the modem on my own. This is my special "gift." Therefore, I was not able to experiment with treatment using a "Rife Machine" – a machine that produces low energy waves used in treatments for those with cancer and other conditions, and used to find the frequency of a condition, sending an impulse of the same frequency to kill or disable the diseased cells. My electro-sensitivity is the reason I couldn't be treated by it (Cancer Research UK, 2018), particularly disappointing, as the Rife Machine works for many people diagnosed with Lyme disease as well and is undergoing more research into its potential uses and responses.

The scientist who invented the Rife Machine believed that all pathogens have vibrations, and if you can attack a pathogen with sound waves - at a higher vibration than the pathogen itself - all pathogens involved in a disease will be destroyed, without damage to the rest of the body. The sound waves enter the body through the hands or feet. Modern day Rife Machines offer "killing" frequencies as well as "supportive" or "healing" frequencies, meaning they can both destroy pathogens *and* support the body in such areas as general healing and collagen-building. For this reason, some consider the Rife Machine a virtual medicine cabinet. It can be used as a singular Lyme treatment or in conjunction with other Lyme disease treatments. Since Rife is not immune-modulating (unlike some herbs and supplements), the machine can be a suitable option for those who have the autoimmune component of Lyme disease. Many patients with Lyme disease who have undergone Rife Machine treatment have reported a strong Herxheimer reaction, meaning a short-term (from days to a few weeks) detoxification reaction in the body.

Science supported the fact that extra electricity existed in my body. My PET scan revealed that my glutamate level (discussed in Chapter 8) was off the chart. I could quite literally *feel* Wi-Fi, Bluetooth (anything that sends out positive charge), and if I stayed near it too long, the burning in my brain became so intense that it felt like I was attached to a light socket. As a result, I would stutter and place my hands on my neck and head to try to keep my thoughts functioning normally. The doctor even asked my husband how many cell phones I had "blown up" due to the overwhelming glutamate levels the electrical forces were causing. I had felt like a total freak up to that point, and since then, I have run into many others afflicted by electro-sensitivity dilemmas. I have had great joy in assuring them that they are absolutely not freaks. It is such a relief!

When your body is in fight or flight mode due to the prominent levels of electromagnetic fields, which can occur due to stress on the central nervous system, the body reacts. Glutamate levels are elevated. The body sends off an electric signal that triggers any electrical functions of devices near the body. I wear my "Q link" device every day to block electromagnetic fields. Keeping myself feeling protected from any external triggers was necessary not only to sleep at night, but to ward off extra distractors that I may not have been aware of.

A cranial sacral massage therapist who was working with a family's infant reached out to me about the baby not being able to sleep in the crib in the room. The baby was crying with no relief. After our discussion, I asked if the crib was close to the wall near an outlet. In fact, it was! I advised the therapist to have the family pull the crib 4 feet away from the wall. They reported back that this was a great solution, and the baby experienced more comfort at night.

I keep a *Qi Shield* device next to my bed every night. It stays in place to protect against EMF radiation and against 5G, while covering a space of 16 x 16 feet out and 6 feet up and down. It is known to work by creating an electrical charge that actually discharges negative ions to counterbalance from the inside of the device. The solution inside releases free electrons, increases the improvements of sleep and decreases EMF radiation. The important thing about this device is that it is not rechargeable and lasts 8 years before it decreases in its power to protect.

> If you or someone close to you have an ongoing difficulty wearing jewelry due to its becoming corrosive, it is a sure sign that your body harbors a high electric field. Have a progressive EMF expert help you prevent EMF illness.
>
> Brian Clement, PhD, LN.

My children didn't understand why we were the only family that did not have Wi-Fi at home. In order to resolve our situation with their homework from school, the goal was to complete the homework with limited exposure to the damaging rays of electromagnetic fields. They retrieved the homework on their laptops using the hotspot on their phones, turned it off while working, turned it back on to submit their assignments, then immediately turned off the hotspot.

On speaking engagements, visiting retirement communities, and meeting with people who experience the same things, I would share the aspects of sleeping and the role electric fields play. Many of the elderly in these communities have difficulty sleeping at night, and the electromagnetic fields are largely to blame. With all of the high frequency charges illuminating from the Wi-Fi and other electrical devices, it is no wonder the residents are not getting their full night's rest. This is an important topic that may be overlooked in many areas of our daily lives. You may find it helpful to explore your level of sensitivity if you have experienced any of these things.

Chapter 5

Liquid Courage

Thinking of numbing your own pain? Do you think it will make things better for you? It's hard to do things on your own strength when you're in a vulnerable state. This is what our emotions tell us when we have reached a breaking point. Tired of the same cycle of trying to ease your mind? While trying to control fears of not getting better, it mentally builds up in the mind and makes things harder to fight off on your own. These "quick fixes" actually stifle you from moving forward in achieving a new you in a greater fashion. For some it may be alcohol and for others it may be a drug. Some people feel the need for excessive shopping, gambling, or anything that will steer the mind from their current reality.

When the pain is so overwhelming, one might do anything to try to get rid of it. I did. Looking for things that will ease the pain can seem like the right way out. We think that by masking the internal conflict with substances, things, or relationships, we can get more relief. This is not the solution.

Pain is nature's and the universe's way to alert us to a need for change and should be acknowledged, not silenced.

Brian Clement, PhD, LN.

45

There are many choices we can make to deal with the woes of pain. It may be returning to something that was once a dependency or even a place of familiarity and comfort. Prescription drugs would not kill the pain for me. So, vodka was my choice of relief and release on some afternoons. It made me feel numb, giving me "liquid courage" to accomplish things I could not do while living in pain. It took the force of pain away. The way I felt closer to normal was by having two short glasses of vodka, soda, and an orange slice. That was my preferred drink - nice and refreshing.

I can't tell you if the drinking was to numb physical pain from the disease, or to numb the mental, physical and emotional pain caused by my husband's withdrawal when it all became too much for him to handle. No one in the family wanted to deal with the crisis which haunted me for years, actually still does. To this day I sometimes reach over in the middle of the night to make sure Darby is still there. The panicked feeling of life without him feels like a recurring nightmare.

The initiative-taking, energetic, and uplifting mother I had always been was struggling way beyond the visible signs. I was hurting my family while I was eliminating my personal pain. I was desperately trying to get to a place of no pain and just peace. I wanted to relieve the pain and sleep at night. I took sleep medications to help me sleep. At the time, I weighed only around 110 pounds, but with these medications, I started gaining weight. All twenty-two pounds came from the negative side effects of some of the medications. It felt that nothing else was working for me. I just wanted relief.

I was raised with parents who would have a cocktail every day at 5:00, so I thought I was just moving into the way I was raised. Generations in my family were cocktail drinkers. According to my friends, this is what their parents did as well, so it must have been that generation! This was another form of "normality" in my reality.

You may be questioning after reading all of this, what was my breaking point? What was the thing that finally brought me to my knees and challenged me to give up the things that I depended on for relief? We all have that "aha!" moment that puts our back up against the wall or causes us to question everything we have done. It is a moment that says "enough is enough." It took a deep self-examination to see my own worth and value, and to know that I was not alone. I had to confront what I had dismissed all along. Help was on the way.

Reluctant and angry, I checked myself into a rehab center. My reaction to the drugs they prescribed for me for alcohol withdrawals affirmed that they were trying to treat a problem that didn't actually exist. What an emotional rollercoaster! I never considered myself an alcoholic; I just knew that I needed to be able to sleep well at night without having a cocktail in the evening or sleeping meds at night. This process shook me to my inner core. There were times in treatment that I regretted walking through those doors. I did not see myself like the others in there nor did I feel that I belonged. Sleepless nights occurred with my mind tossing and turning, questioning how my family and friends were feeling about me and the thoughts of how I got there constantly running through my mind.

This message is not to bring judgment on anyone who has struggled with alcohol or other substances, but to bring awareness that you are not alone in this journey. There is help and this chapter is meant to challenge you to face those inner struggles and become free from any obstacle that is standing in your way. I did it, and so can you.

Chapter 6

Treatment and Healing

Healing can be expressed as a transforming reaction to a foreign adversity that has altered one's life, that returns the body to a healthy state. Whether it's an injury to the physical body or an internal or emotional scar resulting in loss or damage, the body responds to healing as a true beacon of hope. Our bodies respond to an array of treatments in peculiar and fascinating ways, and each individual's healing is designed to help move them forward to health and wellness.

> We are all constantly healing from either an emotional, physical or spiritual concern. This is the natural state that begins at birth and ends at our demise. Be aware and open to the continued process of change that life offers.
>
> Brian Clement, PhD, LN.

In the next phase of my life, I realized that whatever doctors I worked with would need to be "outside the box" thinkers. We needed to heal my immune system, in addition to managing my pain. So, I met with a doctor in Oldsmar, Florida, in 2018, who required a PET scan of my brain (see images on page 75), along with other tests, before our first meeting. This clinic was completely different. From the resolute staff to the knowledge the doctor exuded, all was spectacular in my eyes. I witnessed numerous patients come in from all over the world. They were hoping and believing that they had finally arrived at a place where their questions would be answered.

A precise regimen was put in place for each patient. Protocols were carefully planned that were vital for healing and recovery. There were many areas within my physical body that had already undergone immense treatment, and I could not afford to miss my chance to see what the end would be. Many protocols that a number of physicians presented during various treatments were in hopes they would cure my physical ailments. Yet some were so harsh on my body that these treatment plans were doing more internal damage than good. So, the ultimate goal was to get the body to run on a high octane and understand what the body makes, then add more of it.

It was necessary to see what was functioning in my tissues and organs. The doctor in Oldsmar could read a PET (Positron Emission Tomography) scan and diagnose accurately what was occurring in a patient's organs, specifically the brain. These keen interpretations would determine the types of treatment I would need. This exam uses a radioactive drug (tracer) to show the activity of disease. Any abnormality can be detected on the scan before it shows on other imaging tests.

The doctor's unique formula was a combination of Vitamin C, phosphatidylcholine, amino acids, often an antibiotic, and glutathione - typically the last treatment received - that would cleanse my system. Anti-inflammatories were also needed to rebuild the immune system, along with 800mg of magnesium. My bloodwork was sent to a lab on a weekly basis. I went to colonics more than a couple times a week, and took round-the-clock supplements.

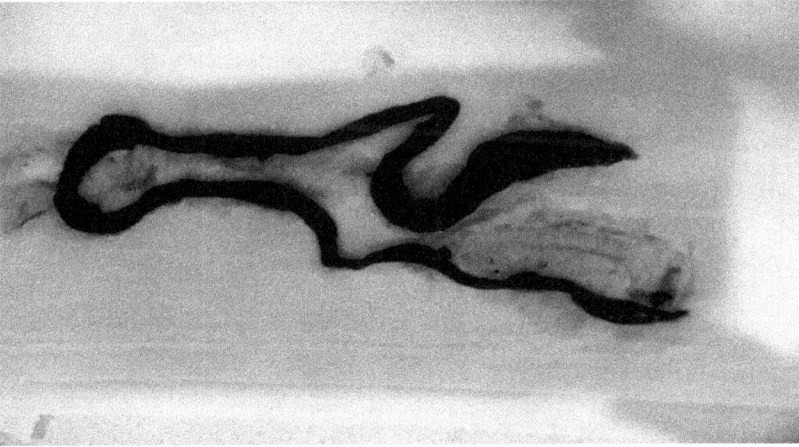

The above image is a parasite a patient expelled (through a bowel
movement) while in Oldsmar undergoing cleansing.
She estimates the overall length was about 3.5 inches.

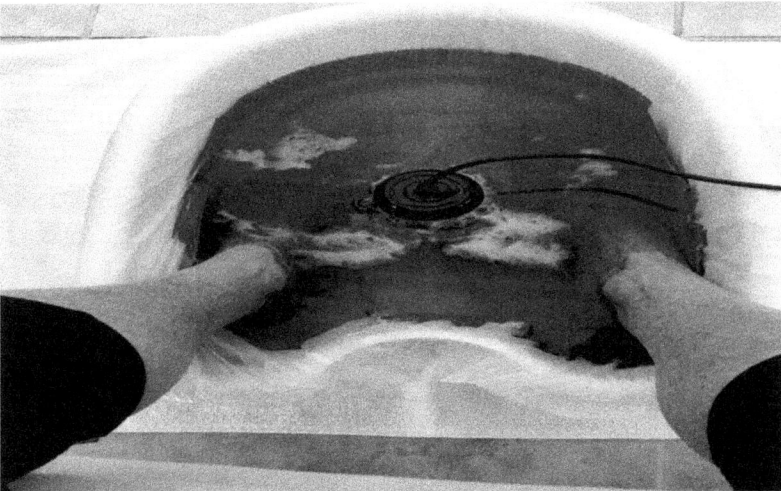

The Ionic Foot Bath is a saltwater bath that uses negative ions
to cleanse the body of toxins. The ions attach themselves to the
toxins and then are flushed out through the feet.

> This ionic foot bath uses electrolysis generating both positive (+) and negative (-) charge. This therapy has the potential to stimulate foot cells and nerves that purges unwanted debris via the large pores of the feet.
>
> Brian Clement, PhD, LN.

The greatest infection was on the left side of my brain, which caused numbness in my left hand. This was also related to my balance issues that would cause me to fall on many occasions. In fact, a few years ago, on an escalator at the Atlanta airport, I fell backwards (thankfully, some men on the escalator caught my luggage and helped me up). I did not even realize I had seriously injured myself. It was not until late in the evening that I noticed my shin bone was exposed! Talk about numbness from real pain – I was physically hurt and did not feel a thing!

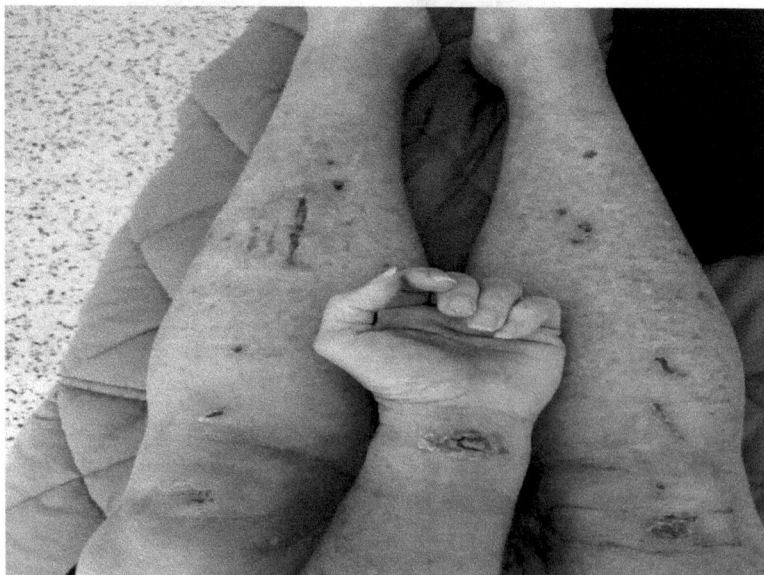

Later, under the same doctor's care, I underwent stem cell treatments - 7 total over a 7-week period. The first three elicited a positive response. After the second treatment, six hours later, I began to experience a "raindrop" feeling in my brain that alleviated the burning sensation. The third treatment brought a level of clear-headedness after I woke up in the mornings - something I had not experienced in years!

Conscious practitioners attempt to clear the body and mindset of health adversaries so that homeostasis and healing occurs.

Brian Clement, PhD, LN.

In hindsight, I should have stopped there, because I didn't feel improvement after the fourth stem cell treatment. I should have allowed my body to rest and absorb the cells before continuing. While no harm was done, treatments four through seven were an unnecessary waste of time and money. I am sure many of you can relate to this scenario: we want speedy results after a rigorous treatment. We need to learn to listen to our bodies when they are trying to tell us what they need to heal.

I recall a time I had left treatment and stopped at a gas station, and I forgot to take out the gas hose - it went with me after I pulled off! Now there you go...so depleted that I needed a real gas of energy! Needless to say, going through rigorous treatments is draining. This is why I recommend having someone by your side at all times - if you are able to.

Through all I had endured, the doctor was extremely impressed by the test results he was seeing. Every physician needs a model of healing to represent what they are doing, and he was encouraged enough to let his patients know the protocols and treatments employed that were making a difference on me. He sent out an email to a majority of his patients that included (with permission) my personal cell phone number. My testimony was that after a few stem cell treatments, my body started to heal significantly. He shared with me that my healing experience gave greater hope to many patients. After the release of his email, my phone rang around the clock. A total calculation of my well-being was up for display. People wanted to see how we did it, what it took, and if it could work for them as well. Testimonials are incredibly important for the journey of progress - that's one of the main reasons for this book.

From doctors with whom I had consulted, to clinics I had visited, the word was out that I had been "cured," or at the very least, I'd gotten some real help. Because of the myriad traditional and non-traditional treatments I had undergone, it became difficult to point to any one thing that gave ultimate healing. I had tried anything and everything to alleviate the pain and re-enter life. To this day I still get calls related to patients with Parkinsons, Alzheimers, dementia, and the like, now even COVID-19, wanting to know how to rebuild an immune system that can truly heal.

Chapter 7

Fungus Among Us

Mold is a separate issue from Lyme disease; it can cause many other diseases and attack the central nervous system. In 2007, a friend asked me if I'd ever had my breast implants checked for mold. At the time I'd had them for ten years, the mark at which people say they can "go bad." So I had a highly acclaimed doctor in Atlanta check them, and we decided I would have them explanted. During the surgery, she discovered that the left implant indeed had mold! While trying to excise the implant, it ruptured, spilling its contents into the cavity, further exposing my system to mold. To make matters worse, I woke up the next morning with a large hematoma which likely indicated blood vessel damage, which would result in more exposure to the bloodstream, and at a faster rate. It's probable that the mold exposure was far greater than it would have been if it had stayed intact.

Upon returning home, I did everything I could to build my immune system, and didn't understand why I wasn't functioning at 100%. A pattern had developed. I would go to a healing clinic for Lyme, receive treatment from exceptional doctors, clean out and boost my system by juicing, experience some relief, then return home only to begin to feel sick again within a few days. *What was I doing wrong?* I had no idea how prevalent the mold inside me was, or that my home was riddled with it.

A blood smear (test showing any abnormalities in red and white blood cells and platelets) in May 2018 opened another Pandora's box. Irregular shapes (termed as ratcheting) on the exterior of my red blood cells showed that mold had entered my bloodstream, and spirochete (serious pathogens that cause diseases in humans) existed in the red blood cells.

Test Name	Result	Units	Flag	Reference Range

Diagnosis 780.79 Fatigue
Diagnosis 782.1 Rash
Diagnosis 780.8 Hyperhidrosis

Special Stains — Run by: ASH on 3/10/2009 4:31 PM
88342 Special Stains (1)

Notes: Many coccobacilli adherent to erythrocytes indicated by arrow(s). This is suggestive of Hemobartonella or Mycoplasma.

In this image from 2009, notice the rough edges of some of the cells, which, if healthy, would be rounded. The cells with the rough edges indicate ratcheting, which is mold.

To view this image in color and for a further description, scan the QR code at the end of the book or go to www.silentkillersbook.com/resources which will take you to my website where you will find multiple color images and other helpful resources.

All because of a spider or tick bite, we needed to eradicate the parasite, treat the inflammation, fight the infection, and remove the mold. Its ferocious and hidden dangers had affected my entire family. In my home, mold was found in the guest room closet. We had to bulldoze half of our home and rebuild.

I would not have known mold's causes in the human body until my test results were revealed years later. Even during this time, my health was challenged in ways I could not imagine. The Biofilm, a thin surface of bacteria that encases itself on substances within the body, protects the mold once it invades your system, and the spirochete attaches itself to the biofilm and makes its own home. It is extremely hard to rid your body of both the pathogen and the mold. Mold is a bigger issue than anyone realizes. It can make you crazy as it is harmful and toxic. It grows and causes a distinct odor in your home from excessive moisture.

Fungus and its related mold is an essential lifeform that in a forest ties together all foliage and trees. In manmade dwellings where one or more of the fungal strains reside and are not symbiotically in harmony with a natural process, the isolated overgrowth is noxious to humans.

Spirochete is a type of bacteria that displays a spiral shape. This family provokes everything from periodontal disease to Lyme and one form even creates syphilis. Its unique ability to ream itself into your cells makes it a formidable and difficult disorder to purge.

Brian Clement, PhD, LN.

57

	Organic Acids Test - Nutritional and Metabolic Profile				
Metabolic Markers in Urine	Reference Range (mmol/mol creatinine)		Patient Value	Reference Population - Females Age 13 and Over	

Intestinal Microbial Overgrowth

Yeast and Fungal Markers

#	Marker	Reference Range		Patient Value	
1	Citramalic	≤ 3.6		2.3	2.3
2	5-Hydroxymethyl-2-furoic	≤ 14		7.4	7.4
3	3-Oxoglutaric	≤ 0.33		0	0.00
4	Furan-2,5-dicarboxylic	≤ 16		4.6	4.6
5	Furancarbonylglycine	≤ 1.9		0.72	0.72
6	Tartaric	≤ 4.5		2.5	2.5
7	Arabinose	≤ 29	H	47	47
8	Carboxycitric	≤ 29		17	17
9	Tricarballylic	≤ 0.44	H	0.53	0.53

Bacterial Markers

10	Hippuric	≤ 613	H	1496	1496
11	2-Hydroxyphenylacetic	0.06 - 0.66		0.34	0.34
12	4-Hydroxybenzoic	≤ 1.3		0.71	0.71
13	4-Hydroxyhippuric	0.79 - 17		13	13
14	DHPPA (Beneficial Bacteria)	≤ 0.38	H	0.84	0.84

Clostridia Bacterial Markers

15	4-Hydroxyphenylacetic (C. difficile, C. stricklandii, C. lituseburense & others)	≤ 19		13	13
16	HPHPA (C. sporogenes, C. caloritolerans, C. botulinum & others)	≤ 208		115	115
17	4-Cresol (C. difficile)	≤ 75		1.4	1.4
18	3-Indoleacetic (C. stricklandii, C. lituseburense, C. subterminale & others)	≤ 11		11	11

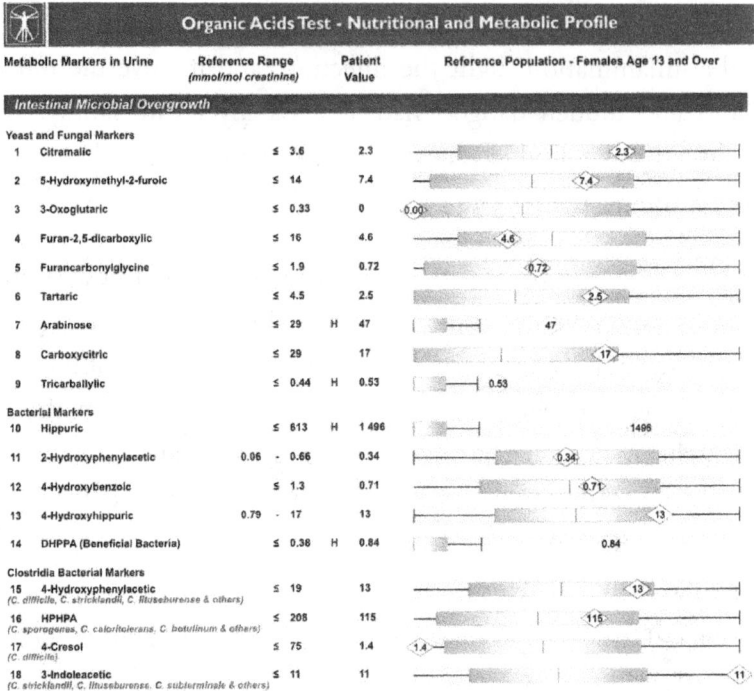

Testing performed by The Great Plains Laboratory, Inc., Lenexa, Kansas. The Great Plains Laboratory has developed and determined the performance characteristics of this test. This test has not been evaluated by the U.S. FDA; the FDA does not currently regulate such testing.

For four consecutive weeks in 2018, my urine was tested for various markers - yeast & fungal, bacterial and Clostridia bacterial.
Above is the result of the fourth week.
You can see my levels were very high in several categories.

To view this image in color and for a further description,
scan the QR code at the end of the book or go to
www.silentkillersbook.com/resources which will take you to my website
where you will find multiple color images and other helpful resources.

I always stayed at the same hotel when I was in town for treatment at the clinic. Especially in humid Florida, hotels have a challenge keeping moisture levels low, which means that mold can be present. The management at the Holiday Inn Express in Dunedin allowed me to have rooms tested to ensure I would be staying in a room that was safe for me. They set things up for me whenever I called, and ensured I had the same room each visit. Nights after leaving the clinic, I would be so depleted that it was all I could do to drive back to the hotel. They were aware that I needed to feel comfortable and secure. They would order dinner for me and have it delivered - their main priority was my ease. They made me feel loved and special every time I walked through the doors.

Fast forward to the summer of 2023 as I was just weeks away from launching this book. I was concerned as some mold symptoms were returning: joint pain, confusion and foggy brain. I had to step outside my house if I wanted to accomplish anything that required actual thinking. So I decided to add ionizers to my A/C system at home after reading reviews which stated that air ionizers purify the air in the room by electrically charging air molecules. They use ions to remove the particulates, microbes and odors from the air. I read that these ionizers kill airborne viruses such as coronavirus which, as you may recall, triggered my relapse in 2022. I didn't know that I once again had mold in my body, so naturally I didn't realize that the weird mold symptoms I was again experiencing were because of the ionizers which were attacking it.

My poor A/C company got my wrath when I read them the Riot Act over the reaction my body was having, but the fact is that without the impact of the air ionizers they installed, I wouldn't have known the mold was present.

Affixing O3 light oxygen devices to your home or office air handler helps destroy mold spores. Most competent air conditioning experts can install these for a low cost.

Years ago I started following an interesting doctor named Todd Farney on his social media sites. He is an expert in the Gut-Brain Axis and its relationship to chronic illness. He works to eliminate chronic illnesses by taking a systems approach. He understands that when addressing his client's ill health, the gut and brain are the epicenter of the problem. His "short clips" of knowledge were subjects that I completely identified with. All of his educating posts covered topics of complex disorders that I had experienced.

I prayed for quite some time about meeting him and the day finally arrived to have that opportunity. A few unusual things happened during my first appointment with him. The Holy Spirit confirmed to me that I was at the right place, at the right time with the right person. The steady stream of tears I had while talking to him came from the affirmations in my heart. I asked him to pen his approach to chronic illness for my readers.

Todd Farney, D.C.

Chronic illness represents a complex array of symptoms that limit activities of daily living and can severely reduce the quality of life for those who suffer from them. Successful recovery requires a holistic perspective of the body to apply multiple behavioral changes, treatment modalities, nutrition, immune support, detox, and healthy communication of all the cells of the body. Taking a shotgun approach and expecting one simple treatment modality to eliminate the problem is ineffective and lacks an understanding of the complexity and intelligence of the body. When you understand that healing comes from above down, inside out, and that the body was created to live and adapt to our environment, you will have a better understanding of how to solve this complex problem.

A typical treatment approach would start with getting as much data as possible about the case for the client that presents for help. We start with a full blood workup and an Organic Acid Test to look at gut microbes, Neurotransmitters, nutritional deficiencies, and the microbiome. In addition, we may use DNA testing, stool analysis, Urine Mycotoxin and mold tests or the DUTCH test to evaluate hormone imbalances. We may choose one or all of these labs to evaluate what is going on. Then, we will do a full consultation and examination to help us understand the complexities of the case. After assessing and finding patterns of dysfunction, we will begin to build a treatment protocol that is customized to each client.

In my practice we have one ultimate goal and three major goals for each client. The ultimate goal is for the client to not need any more help from us. This would mean that they have arrived at a place of health that allows them to do things that they have not been able to do because of their illness. This would also mean that they have the endurance to do such tasks without crashing or having a flare up. The three major goals are: 1) To improve the communication systems of the body so that every cell is communicating with every other cell and to allow for more efficient adaptation, 2) To decrease the load that is a burden to the system, be it toxins, microbes, traumas or inefficiencies, and 3) To empower the client with as many energy resources as possible to accomplish the work that must be done.

I start by establishing healthy digestion and elimination, and then can then move to other areas. Those areas might be empowering the immune system and helping the autonomic nervous system to be in the right balance. After that, I can begin to address deficits, detox difficulties, immune challenges and trauma-induced inability to adapt to life. Using my training in functional and biological medicine, and some specialized tools such as direct resonance testing, I am often able to find solutions for many chronic, complex health conditions.

During my first visit he asked me if I knew that I had AFIB (Atrial Fibrillation), and if I could feel my heart flip-flopping from the severe arrhythmia. My response was that if he could get the buzzing to stop in my head and my feet, maybe I would be able to feel a flip-flop. I told him that, as a matter of fact, if he could get the buzzing to stop and the joint pain to go away, I would run around the building and do a cartwheel. Two weeks later, after being detoxed from mold, the arrhythmia and joint pain were gone. He successfully got my heart back into a normal rhythm. As promised, I ran around the building and did a cartwheel, which he videoed.

I went home with my prescribed tinctures, toxin binders and supplements. My home's mold remediation had begun and I started to not feel like an alien! for a while....

Our house was first treated for mold 14 years ago. Back then, the remediation process was basically to throw everything in the dumpster. We now know that the PVC glue the plumbers used in 2009 slowly rotted over time. In early 2023, when our local electric company replaced our old meter with a new, smaller meter, they didn't properly seal the electrical box on the exterior of our house, and water was able to get into the walls. Serious damage was done in five different areas of our home. We had to hire a mold testing company, a remediation company, a contractor, insulation and air conditioning companies to get our home tested, treated and put back together. This meant months of expenses, stress and living somewhere else. Fortunately we were able to escape both the Florida heat and the mold mess at our home for part of that time in Maine, which we do every summer.

When we arrived in Maine, which had had a rainy summer, what do you think we found at our home there? You guessed it. Think it's a stroke of very bad luck or a super unfortunate coincidence that in both of my homes, mold was discovered at the same time? I don't. I believe far more homes and buildings are crawling in mold, causing a host of mysterious illnesses that should be, but rarely are, attributed to mold.

There was mold all around, but in greatest amounts in the first floor bedroom. As there are far too few remediation companies in Maine, I had to eradicate that mold by myself. The Florida mold remediation company told me what I needed to purchase, and recommended products from a company called Superstratum: the wipe down solution, the fogging supplies and the "sealing" solution. I'm so extremely sensitive to mold that I knew to wear full protective gear: 3mil glove protection, 3M performance respirator, protective goggles and a full-coverage protective suit.

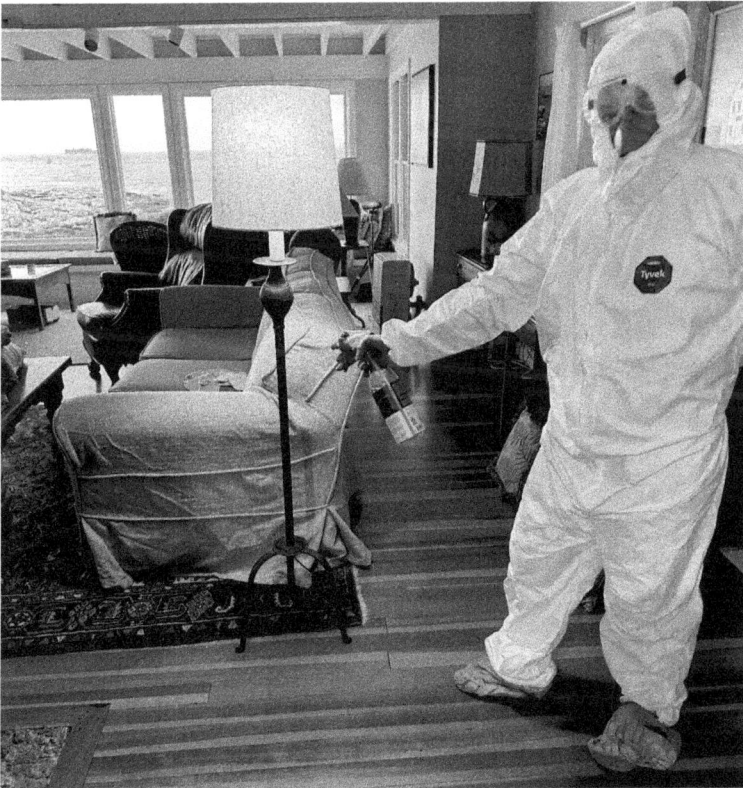

According to Superstratum's website, "By only removing active mold, you leave behind the sticky and dangerous mycotoxins – which can remain for years, wreaking havoc on your health. The latest medical research suggests that mycotoxins, a by-product of mold, can cause devastating chronic inflammation, leading to auto-immune disease in at least 25% of the population. Traditional mold remediation is often not effective in eradicating homes of these toxins. These elusive toxins can hide within walls, under carpets, and in other hard-to-reach areas, making them resistant to conventional cleaning approaches. Moreover, without a comprehensive mycotoxin detox solution, it can quickly regrow and produce harmful mycotoxins again – perpetuating the cycle of health risks for inhabitants."

To keep the mold from returning, it's important to use the proper cleaning products on an ongoing basis to prevent its growth. There are many companies, Superstratum included, which have effective treatments and products.

Brantley May, Indoor Environmental Scientist

The undeniable truth is that all testing methods have their limitations. Air sampling, chemical testing, swab testing, dust analysis and other methods all can provide misleading or incomplete information, especially when applied improperly. Do you notice any unusual odors? Have there been any past water leaks? Amazingly, with the right questions, many issues can be resolved without resorting to any testing at all.

Only a qualified professional with a deep understanding of building science can provide the insight you need about where problems exist and how extensive they are. When seeking the right indoor environmental professional, prioritize hiring a detective – someone who values investigation and doesn't view testing in black and white terms. This approach minimizes the risk of spending thousands on testing and still being left with unanswered questions and no clear direction. Your home is your sanctuary, a place of healing. Finding the right person to diagnose and resolve its issues is crucial.

My contact at Pure Maintenance Mold Remediation in Florida explains well how detection and removal work:

Spencer Zeyer, Pure Maintenance of Jacksonville

A typical project starts with mold detection. This involves visually inspecting the property and the HVAC unit. If you or your family are experiencing allergic reactions that are common from mold exposure, we do some testing. For the initial test, we collect 3 air samples, send them to an independent lab, then go over the results with you. If something needs to be professionally handled, we make a plan to get your home back to a healthy state.

When mold is not disturbed, it will happily eat, drink, and grow. During this "peaceful" time, mold produces mycotoxins, which literally translates to "poison from mold."

When mold is agitated or disturbed, it shoots out spores with the intention of them landing on another habitable surface. There, spores can float for months or even years before landing and starting the growth again. Therefore, containment is key. We must eliminate the possibility of cross-contamination while performing the remediation.

Some experts think one of the factors leading to AFIB are mold mycotoxins. According to Dr. Jack Wolfson in a 2019 article "How Mold Can Cause Atrial Fibrillation," here are several ways that mold can lead to AFIB:

1. Mycotoxins interfere with vitamin D receptors. Vitamin D affects every cell and function in the body. Low vitamin D level is linked to atrial fibrillation. FYI, sunshine lowers AFIB and stroke risk.

2. Mycotoxins are known to interfere with glutathione production and the production of superoxide dismutase and catalase. All of these help with lowering inflammation and oxidative stress. Inflammation is highly linked to atrial fibrillation. Having an ablation? Reducing inflammation can improve success by 76%. Get tested for inflammation AND mold mycotoxins. Inflammation can be from leaky gut. Leaky gut can be from mycotoxins!

3. Mycotoxins impact mitochondrial function. These little fuel factories inside the cell create energy as ATP (anti-tachycardia pacing) and make cellular water. Your heart needs ATP (the "molecular unit of currency" of intracellular energy transfer) to prevent AFIB.

4. Mycotoxins interfere with nitric oxide production. Nitric oxide (NO) keeps blood vessels open. Think nitroglycerin, the pharmaceutical that opens blood vessels and drops blood pressure. This can't happen when mycotoxins are around. High blood pressure is often associated with atrial fibrillation, so we need nitric oxide. NO also helps prevent blood clots.

5. Mycotoxins lead to cellular apoptosis. Could heart cells be dying, thus leading to AFIB?

Mycotoxins interfere with actin. Actin is a protein found in all heart muscle cells. Interfere with the actin, wind up with AFIB.

It's necessary to rid both your home *and* your body of mold. You've read the great lengths I've gone to have a mold-free living environment. To cleanse my body of the toxicity, I eat super-clean and super-green. And I hydrate like crazy.

When my body is inflamed from mold, it's also more sensitive to EMF, which I discussed in great detail in Chapter 4. See how interwoven these sneaky silent killers are?

Scan the below QR code or go to www.silentkillersbook.com/resources for websites of various health providers and book contributors, and for Jennifer's Helpful Health Hacks.

Chapter 8

Science Works

In order for there to be a treatment plan, a diagnosis is required. But you can start doing things even now without a diagnosis as you are going through the search process. Here are some things that will never fail you: get fresh air on a daily basis, go for short walks, clean up your diet, and juice your favorite vegetables. The mountain you are facing won't seem as tall if you have already taken steps to decrease toxins and replace them with good nutrients. You are already supporting your immune system by eliminating toxins as you prepare for results of tests that will be more easily managed.

I have undergone tests and different treatments from doctors all over the world. There were certainly times that I questioned if anything worked at all, or if I was just spinning my wheels. I was spending a lot of money - much of it on erroneous answers and no results. But I now know that all of my experience was for greater purposes – which brings me to this point today. It is necessary to share this informative chapter with you on some of the details that outlined my healing journey.

How many people do not know what to be tested for, and how many physicians have failed to see the signs of an underlying issue? Now with more research, having persistence in caring for your health, and finding people who are willing to speak out on the factors of the unknown, the awareness is becoming greater. All the physicians truly tried their best to get me well; the success of the various treatments had much to do with being able to interpret the Lyme data.

It is pertinent that my readers feel and understand that achieving your healing goal will not always be easy, affordable or enjoyable. Healing is a discovery, and thankfully testing is available using various measures for assessing, understanding, and furthering research for the next generation. I pray that you open yourself to see that there is more opportunity to venture through than just what the doctors say to you regarding your body. Take what they say *and* learn as much as you can for your overall improvement. So, let us get right into the different areas of testing that I underwent, the labs responsible for delivering the results, the definitions of these tests and their descriptions, as well as the effects of the findings.

Blood and urine tests were given weekly while I received infusions. The results showed what toxins (antigenic poisons which are typically derived from microorganisms) were being released and what needed to be treated. It is like peeling an onion. As you take off each layer, the next layer would be the point that treatment would focus on. For example: getting rid of the outer layer of the mold film would possibly reveal Babesia. It was important to see my continued progress or if there was a decline when these tests were done every week. They were then reviewed by my assigned nurse. My chart was reviewed with the physician when red flags were raised and would result in alternate treatment routes. Detection measures taken were key to seeing my blood work results for comprehensive metabolic levels, clotting factors, the purging of any parasites, pathogens, or foreign substances, and any hidden bacterial infections.

Urine analysis testing was sent to Doctor's Data for neuro-biogenic amines, comprehensive amino acids, and toxic metals, as well as toxic and essential elements (packed red blood cells) and DNA methylation pathway profile (whole blood). The Great Plains Laboratory, Inc., was instrumental in assessing a few mycotoxins that revealed *Aflatoxin* (produced by mold species Aspergillus, which are carcinogenic substances in the environment), and *Ochratoxin* (nephrotoxic, immunotoxic, and carcinogenic toxins that are produced by molds in the Aspergillus and Penicillium families). The lab also provided toxic non-metal chemical profiling on industrial toxicants that are commonly found in the environment and are harmful and toxic. Things like gasoline additives and petroleum, household and personal products, pesticides, plastics, colorless liquids, and other fuels and fertilizers were assessed as well.

Also, through Great Plains Laboratory, a nutritional and metabolic profile called Organic Acids Test was obtained to identify intestinal microbial overgrowth and certain metabolites (oxalate, glycolytic cycle, Krebs cycle, amino acid, neurotransmitters, and pyrimidine). It was important to conduct a comprehensive food allergy test as well, as the treatment protocols included eliminating certain foods from my diet. Dairy, legumes, fruit, grains, vegetables, and other foods were evaluated. Moderate reactions came from candida albicans (yeast) and low reactions resulted from dairy. Elevated levels of candida could have been caused by past infections and its overgrowth in my body which gave rise to other food allergies.

Metabolite	Results (ng/g creatinine)	Common Range of Positive Results		
Aspergillus				
Aflatoxin-M1	0.00	3.5 - 20	▲ 3.5	20 ▲
Ochratoxin A	29.28	4 - 20	▲ 4	20 ▲
Gliotoxin	752.04	200 - 2000	▲ 200	2000 ▲
Penicillium				
Sterigmatocystin	0.00	0.2 - 1.75	▲ 0.2	1.75 ▲
Ochratoxin A	29.28	4 - 20	▲ 4	20 ▲
Mycophenolic Acid	97.86	5 - 50	▲ 5	50 ▲

My MycoTox Profile from 2018

To view this image in color and for a further description, scan the QR code at the end of the book or go to www.silentkillersbook.com/resources which will take you to my website where you will find multiple color images and other helpful resources.

Lyme Disease Data

The Lyme Multi-Peptide IgG Elisa Assay Report has index values that consist of results pertaining to normal ranges of Lyme disease. According to the Immunoscience Lab, the chronic nature of Lyme disease and antigenic diversity of spirochetes, suggest that antigenic variation plays a vital role in immune invasion (Immunoscience Lab, n.d.). As an interjection to the testing performed, though pertinent data and information provided is a factor produced from the Immunoscience lab, the results obtained from this lab are not FDA approved (at the time of this book release). In addition, there is correlation in the bloodwork that is a cross-reaction of the results identified in the blood-stream. The Centers for Disease Control and Prevention recommends the Serologic Diagnosis of Lyme titers (concentration) to detect Lyme disease. This performance uses sensitive enzyme immunoassay (EIA), or immunofluorescence assay followed by western immunoblot assay for specimens yielding positive or equivocal results (CDC, n.d.).

The Lyme peptides that were of most relevance and detected on the Lyme disease panel were examined carefully to see what antibiotics worked best. Babesia *microti* is transmitted by tick bites, typically in the Northeast and Midwest. Due to its infective state, Babesiosis can then infect the red blood cells and spread. It is treatable and preventable. Bartonella infection, also known and related to Cat Scratch Disease (CSD), Trench Fever, and Carrion's Disease, can produce fever, enlarged or tender lymph nodes, headaches, rashes, and pain (CDC, 2019).

Years ago, a feral cat was hanging out underneath my house. Mary Cleary, owner and veterinarian of At Home Veterinary Care, advised me to get rid of the cat, as they are known to carry toxoplasmosis. The disease can be carried in the sand, feces, and urine, or where the cat or animals lay. Therefore, the infected cat would pose a danger by infecting my other pets and/or humans. There was a risk that one or both of my dogs would get infected with the disease.

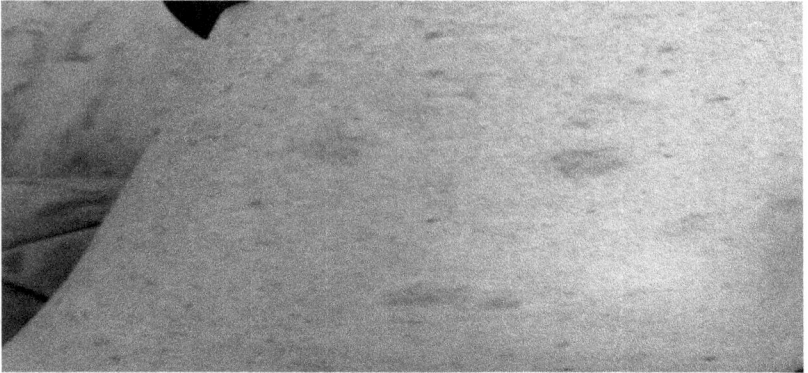

Evidence of Bartonella

Ehrlichia (Ehrlichiosis) is the infection that starts after being infected by a tick. Severe headaches, nausea, confusion, and chills are early symptoms. When progressive, the illness poses critical risk factors associated with brain or nervous system damage, respiratory or organ failure, and can even lead to death if not treated (CDC, 2019). Borrelia *burgdorferi*, a spirochete which is the cause of Lyme disease, is transmitted through the bacteria of ticks, spiders or mosquitoes, which must be infected in order to pass on to humans.

In March of 2018, the initial data retrieved prior to the entrance into the clinic showed that the four peptides previously identified were out of normal range, except for Ehrlichia. Over the course of a couple of months into the treatment, the results of Bartonella on the Lyme multi-peptide assay, showed a significant decrease from when I first entered the clinic. August of 2019 was the last testing on the Lyme data performed prior to the exit of the clinic. It showed an elevated amount of Babesia, and the results were over the normal level for Borrelia.

Positron Emission Tomography (PET)

The PET scan results of March 30, 2018 were the driving force to populate the overall treatment plan. Included in the report were the findings of Lyme disease and Mold Toxicity that had taken their course and caused the illnesses to progress rapidly over time.

The second PET scan, September 27, 2018, was conducted six months into treatment. At this point, the doctor had been heavily treating me with antibiotics, stem cells, supplements, colonic therapy and other efforts to rid my bloodstream of the Lyme and toxins.

To view this image in color and for a further description, scan the QR code at the end of the book or go to www.silentkillersbook.com/resources which will take you to my website where you will find multiple color images and other helpful resources.

In neuroscience, glutamate is the anion (negatively charged ion) of glutamic acid in its role as a neurotransmitter (a chemical that nerve cells use to send signals to other cells). It is by far the most abundant excitatory neurotransmitter in the nervous system and is related to the ability to learn and effectively use cognitive functions. In a "normal" brain, GABA (Gamma-Aminobutyric Acid), another neurotransmitter also found throughout the brain, keeps glutamate in check. The conversion of glutamate to GABA occurs via the enzyme Glutamic Acid Decarboxylase (GAD) and prevents both elevated levels of glutamate and diminished levels of GABA. Simply put, for a healthy brain to function, GABA & glutamate must be in balance. Too much glutamate is a terrible thing for the brain - it can over-excite nerve cells, causing them to die which can become dire over a prolonged period of time. The other side effect of too much glutamate is inflammation.

Additionally, elevated glutamate in the body depletes glutathione, a critical antioxidant. Glutathione prevents damage to important cellular components caused by reactive oxygen species, such as free radicals, peroxides, lipid peroxides, and heavy metals. Glutathione decreases with age, and lower levels have been detected in individuals with cancer, HIV/AIDS, type 2 diabetes, hepatitis, and Parkinson's disease. Symptoms of excessive glutamate in the brain include pain amplification, anxiety, restlessness, insomnia, and ADHD-type symptoms related to focus. Additionally, excess glutamate in response to underlying infection contributes to additional symptoms like obsessive-compulsive disorder (OCD), depression, sleep disturbances, seizures, and tics. All of these symptoms can coincide with Lyme disease.

Oh, and did you know that over 70% of your immune system is in the gastrointestinal tract...which is lined with glutamate receptors? That is something to think about. How do you find out if you have excessive glutamate? The easiest and most cost-effective way to test is by tracking diet changes and watching for behavioral changes. One of the simplest tests to perform is a urine amino acid analysis which provides an overall average of glutamate and GABA levels, but can be unreliable as it is unable to detect if glutamate is pooling in certain areas of the brain (which is often the case). A simple blood test can check blood plasma glutamate levels, but again will offer an overall average instead of a clear picture. Unfortunately, one of the most reliable ways to test for glutamate levels is a lumbar puncture which measures the glutamate levels in the cerebrospinal fluid, which is quite invasive. A brain MRI with a 5 Tesla resolution can offer an indication as to where glutamate is pooling in the brain.

Regardless of testing and its results, lowering dietary exposure to glutamate can help. Gluten, dairy, soy, corn, and processed food should all be avoided. Other foods high in glutamate include nuts, tomatoes, certain sauces (stay away from MSG, aka Monosodium Glutamate), seafood, mushrooms, peas & starchy vegetables. Foods lower in glutamate include green leafy vegetables, seeds, chica, flax, and sesame, herbs such as lemon balm & chamomile, and blueberries.

The following nutrients and nutritional supplements can be instrumental for restoring cognitive function after the body's production of excess glutamate:

1. **Phosphatidylcholine**: a phospholipid that supports the function of many organs, such as the pancreas and liver, and plays a significant role in the transport and metabolism of fats, cell membrane synthesis, and inflammation reduction. It helps make a neurotransmitter responsible for learning, focus, and concentration.

2. **5 HTP**: an amino acid that contributes to the body's manufacture of the neurotransmitter serotonin. Serotonin enhances mood, energy, sleep and digestion but can also assist with memory & cognitive function.

3. **L-tyrosine and L-DOPA:** amino acids that make dopamine, a neurotransmitter that treats low energy, depression, and cognitive dysfunction

4. **L-acetyl carnitine:** an amino acid that can improve cognition and delay Alzheimer's progression.

5. **L-huperzine A:** a compound that preserves acetylcholine in the brain by preventing its breakdown which aids in memory & cognition

6. **Vinpocetine:** a synthetic derivative of the vinca alkaloid vincamine which can increase oxygen and blood flow to the brain and protects it against the effects of glutamate.

> Search out food-derived or food-based supplements that contain cofactors which often facilitate absorption and digestion at a much higher level.
>
> Brian Clement, PhD, LN.

The importance of this section was to highlight factual testing and results that were conclusive to my diagnoses. I felt it necessary to pinpoint crucial pieces of my health journey into the various treatments, to give my readers an alternative route to find an even greater solution. There were clearly things that I did not fully understand scientifically, but I gathered as much information along the way to be able to share it with you. In addition, the types of tests and routines I endured may not be the route for you. I encourage you to take note of these avenues and consult with your physicians on considering their uses, techniques, and strategies for optimal health.

Chapter 9

Health and Wellness

Focusing on your own well-being is crucial not only for yourself, but for ensuring those around you are living their best lives as well. I was heavily involved in my children's activities; health and fitness were integral in our family, and still are to this day. When we started going through illnesses in our home, it caused us to question what was happening. We were living in a sick house that had mold in it. During this time, we could not understand why our middle child, Darby Jr., was having infections so severe they caused him to have three sinus surgeries between the ages of four and six! Jennings had gastrointestinal complications; Kendall had mold markings on her legs that looked like stretch marks (which eventually went away). We were dealing with doctor appointments that were exhausting.

I began to take matters into my own hands. Fitness was an alternative to frustration. This is one of the reasons we mention that exercising is a tool to be grounded with your body, mind, and environment. You begin to experience what is missing, what is needed and how the body responds to danger, stress, and low immunity. Exercise is one of the most beneficial tools of being in tune with your mind when encountering illnesses. Receiving negative doctor reports should propel you to make necessary changes to reverse the findings. Taking authority over your body can give you the confidence that is needed to push you through.

Hyperbaric chambers that are widely accessible will help you saturate your body with oxygen that strengthens immunity, toxins are released and an overall feeling of well-being is gained.

Brian Clement, PhD, LN.

My body loves to sweat! The best investment that I have made was an infrared sauna. It has changed my life over the years, and I have used it to rid my body of unwanted toxins. Infrared saunas have an enormous impact on detox and help in losing weight. The experience of my head feeling clear when I get out is rewarding as well as refreshing. I do three sweat sessions in my time in the sauna. Thermal Life and Jacuzzi Clearlight Low EMF are high-quality brands that have been around for a long time. I lay towels on the floor, and use a towel wrapped around me. Sit on two towels and have three towels to use for the three rounds of sweat sessions. I placed my sauna in the laundry room where it is easily accessible. Make sure you have the largest container of water near you while using the sauna. Staying hydrated is key. A helpful tip: avoid using the same towel for sweating that you use for wiping *off* the sweat which contains the toxins, to aid in a more detailed purification process. By the third round in the sauna, you should be working up to the heat level. Build up the body by detoxing appropriately. The benefit is that toxins are being excreted from the body. The infrared rays go deeper into the cells that excrete through the skin than a regular sauna. I highly recommend getting one for your home if it is affordable for you. Or link up with others who also may benefit and pitch in together. Everyone needs to find out what works for them while using the infrared saunas. Create your own protocol for when to use it on a weekly basis. The key is to eat more healthfully and sweat more.

Saunas create an atmosphere that raises the core body temperature. You sweat, your heart rate increases, and your body pumps more blood to your skin. This is your body's way of cooling down. This process mimics the effects of exercise and provides similar health benefits. Traditional saunas use heating elements to raise the temperature of the air inside. But infrared saunas use infrared light to heat your body, opening up your cells to release toxins deep within.

> Near and far infrared saunas remove 87% more heavy metal and toxic debris than traditional Scandinavian types. Research on paraplegics revealed that they received up to 40% of the benefits gained by aerobic exercise after 20 minutes at the temperature of 140 degrees F. Steam Vapor baths are another option, yet do not remove deep tissue debris as well as the heat therapies. The steam helps lungs, bladder, kidney, and at a lesser level, the overall system.
>
> Brian Clement, PhD, LN.

For me, adding infrared sauna to the Lyme disease treatment plan was advisable because of the detoxification benefits which accelerated the healing process. Infrared heat penetrates deep into the body's organs and tissues detoxifying them through the skin's sweat. Neurotoxins (those which infect nerve cells) released from Lyme disease can cause fever, fatigue, and depression, and if left untreated can affect the joints, heart, and nervous system. Deep penetration of infrared heat can flush neurotoxins out of the body through the skin which is preferable to putting excess stress on the kidneys and liver to eliminate those neurotoxins. Infrared heat is also able to increase blood circulation by penetrating the body's joints, muscles and tissues, allowing more oxygen to circulate to injured areas of the body and reduce inflammation and the pain often associated with Lyme disease.

On a vacation, my kids and I got suited up in our scuba equipment and dove eleven feet in a pond. To my surprise, the barometric pressure and pure oxygen provided a significant relief in pain! I later consulted an internist who had previously served as a Navy pilot, and he completely understood. He wrote me a prescription for 49% nitrogen/51% oxygen, with which I would fill my scuba tank and swim around the bottom of our family's salt-water pool. The pain subsided! When the pain was at its worst, I would often leave work, don the scuba tank, jog on the bottom of the pool for 10 minutes, get out of the pool, re-dress, and then go back to work. Body surfing in the ocean even helped from the standpoint of moving my lymphatic system around and draining toxins from my body. Grounding – also known as earthing – in the sand at the beach, also provided (and still provides) some relief.

Here are a few things that would help me gain the strength, mobility, and mental energy I needed to have a productive day. In the mornings, I would use breathing mechanisms to get the brain working. Who does not want a healthy brain? Incorporating flexibility, spinal flex, abdominal, self-massage, and meridian exercise techniques opened up my senses and cleared my mind for the day.

A remarkably interesting technique that I found to work well is called *tapping*. It is a style of movement that involves using two fingertips and lightly tapping on traditional acupuncture points: between the eyebrows, the thyroid area, the chestplate. Stop for a moment and try it while your eyes are closed. Gently tap those areas as it will awaken your sensory and perception skills. I have heard some people say that these techniques gave them clarity in their work and a brighter start to their day.

> Tapping therapy, also known as Emotional Freedom Technique, was born out of Gary Craig's work and has been studied with positive results at both the University of Michigan and Stanford.
>
> Brian Clement, PhD, LN.

My mother always told me that I was allergic to penicillin and sulfa. One physician I went to actually wanted to give me penicillin *knowing I was allergic to it*, and assured me that if a reaction occurred, he would put a straw in my windpipe to breathe. You better believe I was out of there! Needless to say, I have had my share of encounters with some interesting doctors.

As I searched for other interventions along the way, Body Electronics, taught by Encompass Life, was a great channel of positive energy that kept me going. The teachings provided information on the endocrine system and the power of positive energy. The class was designed to encourage participants to speak positive and powerful words over their bodies. This can influence the body to become strengthened with the power to change the negative effects of disease to a powerful state of healing.

> Body electronics was created by John Whitman Ray. This body/mind therapy combines principles of acupuncture, kinesiology, reflexology and ancient healing practices. Its objective is to resolve physical and emotional blockages.
>
> Brian Clement, PhD, LN.

I strongly recommend that you check out the "Medical Medium" books. The author shares a wealth of information on the food groups that are used for curing diseases. Different ailments in the body are aligned with the necessary foods that can aid in rebalancing the body and providing fuel for longevity and proper nourishment. Educating yourself on the foods you consume is fundamental in preparing your body to fight against foreign substances. In doing this, you will be equipped for the journey to get the best out of your healing through healthier foods.

Healthful eating comes with great discipline and self-control. The first key is training the mind to think about healthful choices and finding ways to enjoy new varieties of foods. Incorporating foods like spinach, mixed lettuces and liquid aminos add complete balances to many meal selections. Think about including foods that are high in vitamins A, K, and D. Ensure that you eat the things that can spoil in 3 days. It may require you to go to the grocery store frequently. Going to the store every 3 days propels me to eat more healthful foods and not waste them. If you feel that you cannot make frequent trips to the grocery store, local fruit, and vegetable stands, try taking advantage of delivery services that will bring the items you need to your home. The goal is to keep your body feeling refreshed with quality foods and making better choices for your diet.

> We share this beautiful planet with at least eight million other species. In nature, they all consume a 100% raw food diet and suffer magnificently less disease. Science today supports the consumption of organic plant food in its uncooked form as the ideal nutrition for health, healing and longevity.
>
> Brian Clement, PhD, LN.

I will never forget the highly intense experience I had at the Kushi Institute in 2007 - a one-week immersion program. Thank goodness my dear friend Suzanne was with me because she was already familiar with the Kushi Institute protocol. To illustrate the level of specificity, we learned the proper way to slice a carrot for optimal nutritional benefit. Same for a cucumber.

Many people who attended this unique place had cancer or other serious conditions. Attendees were placed on a specific diet, which was considered macrobiotic counseling. My major health concerns and diagnoses at this time were toxic metal poisoning, Epstein-Barr, Lyme disease, viral meningitis, headaches, fatigue, allergies, and disturbed sleep. At the time I wasn't even aware I was also battling mold.

I learned so many things that were crucial elements of healing the body through foods. Eating all natural from the garden, chewing food thoroughly to get enough out of enzymes, and preparing my meals properly resulted in the best nutritional value. The goal is to preserve the enzymes in the foods we consume.

In addition to learning the proper way to cut vegetables, it was recommended to add scallions and herbs such as parsley, thyme and cilantro as they are natural detoxes. Adjusting cooking to age and sex, daily activity, and the consumption of 20-30% of vegetables a day, were also helpful tools. I am sure we all know that flour products are not so good for the body. Excluding them from the diet was highly recommended at the Kushi Institute.

It was my first time learning the precise way to heat oil, as olive oil can be ruined as it burns longer. It then becomes carcinogenic. Well, that certainly made me rethink how to use oil when cooking! The foods not recommended were many of the things I loved to eat, but to my surprise, there were recommended foods I had never heard of or thought of eating. Have you ever tried: daikon, somen noodles, mochi, burdock, dandelion root, pattypan squash, or mizuma? We also learned the brilliant uses of incorporating miso into our diets. It aided in building immune system health and strengthening the body.

> Macrobiotics was developed by Micho Kushi who mentored under George Oshawa, a Japanese spiritual philosopher. The diet that Kushi created was loosely based on a traditional ancient discipline. It is often a good first step for those leaving behind a toxic western cuisine. For those who require rapid turn-around, it is best to move into a less processed and purer raw diet.
>
> Brian Clement, PhD, LN.

Juicing food can become your natural medicine. It separates the juice from the fiber of the vegetable and fruit. This is why I recommend adding a juicer to your daily life. It has changed my life dramatically. Fresh stalks of celery have benefited me in so many ways. Upon daily consumption of a cup of celery juice (a natural purifier) on an empty stomach I actually *feel* the enzymes in my lower abdomen, and my brain feels refreshed. The first-time juicing celery, I could not believe the feel of the celery's texture. No wonder it is a vegetable that can be hard to digest for people who have digestive or intestinal issues! My celery juice regimen has opened my eyes to a deeper understanding of eating foods in the proper and more healthful way.

Now that you have had a different tour through my nutritional map, do you ever think about the ingredients in your cosmetics and health care items that go onto the surface of your body? Just another thought to propel you into researching things that may contribute to some of the symptoms you experience. I am only sharing some of this information as it intrigues me because of the officially known harmful effects on humans, yet they are still distributed all around us. It can get pretty deep, and my advice is to not overthink it or live in fear of your normal daily life; just make yourself aware of what goes into and on your body.

Healthy Beauty is the title of a book written by the renowned toxicologist Dr. Epstein. It reveals the endless disease-causing chemicals in cosmetics globally. Many of the so-called "natural" varieties are also filled with harmful ingredients. This is equally important to consider when living a healthy, illness-free life.

Brian Clement, PhD, LN.

Chapter 10

Courage Brings Freedom

Courage is the ability to move forward while being bombarded with the headwinds of negative thoughts and energy. Trying to navigate a transformed life through constant fear, criticism and chastisement, can be a task all by itself.

I created a company, Faceforward Global, LLC when I became an independent consultant for a multi-level marketing company. It also was useful as a parent company for my children's initial businesses, helping them get started on the road to independence. One of the reasons I named my company Faceforward Global is that I felt I was facing a dragon that was trying to devour my health every day. This was a representation of me *facing forward* in all times of trouble. Regardless of my own determination, there were people close to me who surely judged me and my situation. They saw my ups and downs. They saw me fall and get back up again (literally, I would fall on the ground due to my left leg constantly dragging, brush myself off, and get back up). It is easy for people to look critically from the outside. This created a hesitancy to share my feelings or internal concerns with them. It is best to have people near you whom you can truly count on when all hell breaks loose. You will know who is really there for you when you need them the most.

Healing requires patience, understanding, and courage. Courage does not stem from fear, nor does it create an entrapment within us. It takes immense courage to tear down the walls and move forward. Simple activities that were challenging had taken tolls on my physical body. The piece that held me together was *courage*. I became brave and released the fear of falling down every time I was walking. I stared defeat in the eyes and pushed my body to the maximum limit with a conquering attitude. I was no longer afraid of the blood, scabs, and scars. They were all reminders that my healing was actively moving forward.

I have found my voice and in this I try to help as many people as possible by being more straightforward. My depth of compassion is much greater, and my empathy level is much higher than it was before Lyme disease, for which I am grateful. Residual effects still exist, but it is nothing compared to what I experienced in the throes of Lyme and mold.

When it was time to discover healing, the Emotion Code was the avenue that opened the path for me to face my many adversities. The Emotion Code technique, developed by Dr. Bradley Nelson, identifies and releases trapped emotional energy in the body which cause imbalances. Trapped emotions are identified through muscle testing and released by using magnets to balance the body's energy field. It aims to promote healing, improve physical health, relieve emotional distress and enhance overall well-being, and can be used in concert with traditional medical and psychological treatments.

Emotion Code created a gateway that released trapped emotions embedded in my mind and spirit and allowed my body to heal faster and more efficiently. This process of healing also alleviated physical discomfort, eased my emotional wounds, restored relationships, and developed a breakthrough of what was sabotaging me. It also allowed the full discovery, exposure, release, and the ability to empower myself and others through the healing components.

In my healing sessions using the Emotion Code it was identified that I had a thick "wall" around my heart. Burdens were beginning to shed, and the reward came from believing that these emotions existed as a result of events that took place around me that only my subconscious was remembering. These dilemmas needed to be uprooted and dealt with. Things that were still lingering in my life were easily invoked through any stimulation, where residual sins needed releasing. Imbalances were caused by things stored in my mind and prompted me to confront the holding on to negative emotions. The underlying root causes that were blocking growth were also at the forefront of healing my emotions. These were pertinent steps used in the Emotion Code that unveiled what was causing me to die inside while others did not see it. It was worth taking the time to confront the tortured thoughts in my mind that were generated from past experiences I was not even aware of. It was vital to emotionally remove those things that were clinging on to my future. For more information and resources on Emotion Code, go to www.silentkillers.com/resources.

This is what I present to you: the authenticity of my heart. It is time to release all of those negative and toxic emotions today! Find the courage within yourself to keep striving no matter what it looks like. May you see the benefits of emotional and physical healing within.

Part 2: My Healthcare Team

I can't even count the number of people who played significant roles in my long quest for healing. But several had so profound an impact and have so much to offer my readers that I asked them to tell my story from their perspectives.

Chapter 11

As a Health Coach

Michelle Spires

When I met Jennifer in 2015, she was on the hunt for anything that could help her. She had done all of the "normal" things and very little was helping. She had heard from a couple who said that Raindrop Technique had helped them tremendously when she found me.

Raindrop Technique is so powerful because it supports all of the systems of the body simultaneously - immune, digestive, respiratory, circulatory, spinal, nervous - you name it, it's supported. There are specific oils used in a specific order to aid the body on a cellular level. The oils fall into 3 categories: phenols, monoterpenes, and sesquiterpenes. For compliance reasons, you'll have to research these on your own and find out how they operate in our bodies. The oils, partnered with the application process (or technique), also support the body shifting from fight or flight/sympathetic nervous system and return to ease/parasympathetic nervous system. This in and of itself is powerful, as where there is EASE there is no dis-ease. They cannot simultaneously exist. The amount of this shift is directly related to the person's willingness to have ease in their life. For some, their familiar zone is so wrapped into life being hard, tiring, undeserving, or uncomfortable that their shifts take a bit longer. The oils can work in the system for up to a week. Most of my clients measure ¼-1 inch taller after their sessions. The muscles relax and the vertebrae begin to realign. Other testimonials I have gotten from my clients after their sessions include immense relaxation, clear thinking, smooth digestion, increased appetite (someone who was underweight), cleared sinuses, released locked shoulder, restored sleep, and much more.

High-quality, therapeutic grade oils also support us on an emotional level aromatically. They bypass the frontal lobe (the thinking brain) and go straight to the limbic brain through the olfactory nerves. Through the limbic brain they can support us moving through old dramas and traumas that have run us for decades. Many times, during sessions, clients have old memories that come up for healing. I am a life coach, and I use oils to support my clients on a physical and emotional level as they upgrade their health and overall life. I work very closely with the body signals specific to each person to find their roots. Each signal has a different conversation tied to it. Every word, thought, and feeling creates our reality. The common conversation about Lyme begins with "I'm sick and tired of...". At some point, most folks with Lyme said, thought, or felt this or something similar to it. Their subconscious took the directive and went about building it for them by whatever means necessary to have it manifest for them including in their physical body. When we find the source of the conversation, we can reverse it and create something new.

Chapter 12

As an Integrated Holistic Practitioner

Rebecca Leigh Morey

I specialize in alternative healing modalities for balancing the body, mind, and spirit. Empowering people to help themselves with their health and emotional challenges is my passion! There is nothing more rewarding for me than helping a client find relief, peace and to feel better! The specialties that I perform are: Spiritual and Emotional Healing as a Certified Emotion Code Practitioner to Sound Healing, Pranic Healing, Akashic Record Reading, Crystal Healing, Angel Healing, and more. I am delighted to share my experience with Jennifer. I incorporate my Divine intuition, education, and spiritual gifts into all of my work. My passion is to help people release the energies that are no longer serving them.

Jennifer contacted me in June of 2020, reporting difficulty healing from a long battle with Lyme and mold toxicity. We quickly determined that in order to transform Jennifer's health, we had to heal her energy. But first, Jennifer needed to understand how our energy works and the importance of maintaining it for ultimate health. Our bodies are made of energy. Our cells, tissues, blood, hair, and skin are involved in the healing process. Every living thing has energy! Energy flows through our body, tissues, and cells. Without energy, we would not be alive, right?

Within your physical body you have an energy system. This system is made up of seven chakras. "Chakra" means "disk" or "wheel" and refers to the energy centers in your body. These wheels (or disks) of spinning energy are located along the spinal column running from the bottom of your spine to the top of your head. Each area corresponds to certain nerve bundles, major organs, emotions and color. To function at your best, your chakras need to stay open, balanced and energized. If the chakras get blocked, you may experience negative physical, emotional, and energetic symptoms.

A person with any type of autoimmune dysfunction (i.e. Lyme, Lupus, fibromyalgia or mold toxicity), typically shows signs of extremely congested, dirty, and dense energies within the entire chakra system, as well as within their organs, glands, and tissues, more so than the average person. It's as if there were an invisible, toxic smog as thick as molasses. This foreign covering smothers the organs, tissues, and body. In return, it keeps the body polluted, sick, unable to heal, and leaves a person literally feeling stuck in the mud.

Energetically speaking, Jennifer was very dense with dirty energies. The chakras were totally blocked with no flow of energy. It was as if her energies were barely circulating in the toxic smog filled with the energetic residue of the Lyme and mold pathogens. Yuck! We determined quickly that there were many imbalances within her energy system, as well as in her physical body, that were causing these resistances to heal physical and emotional pain, brain fog and low energy. Jennifer and I created a recipe for healing that would propel her further into the next chapter of her health journey:

RECIPE FOR HEALING:

- Emotion Code

- Pranic Healing

- Crystal Healing

- Meridian Alignment

We got to work by having a conversation with Jennifer's subconscious mind (SCM). The SCM stores every single piece of information about *you* since conception. It told us exactly where to find the imbalances and blockages. There were trapped emotions in the organs and glands, lymphatic system, as well as circulating dirty energy within the circulatory system.

Over the course of four months we released, cleaned, corrected, cleared, realigned, and energized every single organ, muscle tissue and chakra that was in disharmony. Emotional blockages in the chakras and subtle energy bodies were cleared, allowing the healing to begin. This type of healing work has allowed Jennifer's subconscious mind to completely release the compounded traumas and trapped emotions she has been carrying her whole life. The invisible emotional baggage had prevented her body from fully being able to heal. Freeing her organs, tissues, chakras, and entire energy body, Jennifer received a release from all of the lower diseased energies; thus, allowing the body to naturally heal as it was intended to do.

As we released the emotional blockages, Jennifer's body started responding positively! It was as if we broke through this invisible barrier that was holding onto the Lyme and mold energies. Finally! Jennifer was able to receive the clean, positive, and energized healing that was needed to flow through her organs, systems, and chakras in order to heal itself!

Jennifer's dedication to put in the time and effort to complete each session was impressive! She was determined to allow the new energies to integrate and make the appropriate shifts the physical body needed to heal. Jennifer released numerous imbalances, inherited emotions, compounded traumas from her childhood, as well as parasitical energetic conglomerates that were trapped in the digestive system. She released psychic traumas, emotional shock energies and hundreds of trapped emotions that were stuck in organs like the spleen, liver, stomach and heart. Jennifer released a "Heartwall" with 68 emotions blocking her healing progress.

Not only am I thrilled for Jennifer's healing success, but I'm also so proud of her! This journey is not for the faint of heart. It's a tough road. Lyme and mold are no joke.

With the combination of releasing the emotional energies and imprints, and cleaning and balancing the chakras, Jennifer embraced her healing progress by releasing the toxic Lyme and mold energies that were keeping her body in disharmony. The results speak for themselves. Her body, mind and spirit are stronger, healthier, happier and free of disharmony and dis-ease.

Chapter 13

As a Physician of Traditional Chinese Medicine

Dr. Chip Sexton AP, DTCM

There are health concerns in modern times that remain elusive to conventional and holistic diagnosticians alike. The rise in complex symptomatology of inflammatory conditions related to Lyme disease and its co-infections, environmental toxicity, and autoimmune diseases can be difficult for healthcare providers to understand and adequately treat, leaving patients with unsatisfying results. As a physician of Traditional Chinese Medicine (TCM), it is common to see patients who have been unsuccessful seeking conventional medical treatment alone. This is a place where TCM shines. However, in cases as listed above, even TCM diagnostics have fallen short until relatively recent times.

The notion of *Gu Zheng*, or ghost syndrome, arose in Chinese Medicine in the 7th century, but has disappeared from the modern practice of TCM in China. Thanks to the efforts of modern scholars of TCM, clinicians now have a better way to understand and treat these complex health issues. According to Heiner Fruehauf PhD, Founding Professor of the College of Classical Chinese Medicine at National University of Natural Medicine, "in general, there is very little aware-ness of what *Gu* Syndrome really is—a chronic inflammatory syndrome, or a super-infection involving lots of different pathogens like funguses, viruses and spirochetes at the same time." (1) "By definition [Gu] is not a regular parasitic infection, but a condition that weakens the entire organism by having become systemic in nature." (2)

Due to an over-administration of antibiotics along with a prevalence of international travel, complex infections are more prevalent today. Overuse of antibiotics can damage the body's microbiome and leave us susceptible to new infections. The prevalence of international travel allows for exposure to parasites on foreign soil. Individuals with parasitic infections transmitted through hand-to-mouth or the fecal/oral route, can bring these infections to other countries as well. Though an initial infection may not present any symptoms, as the immune system becomes overburdened, it struggles to manage subsequent exposure to pathogens. As a result, infection and inflammatory elements wreak havoc on the system leading to a myriad of symptoms which can be difficult to deal with.

Modern TCM consists of five branches of therapeutic practices. The first is Nutrition. Most modern TCM practitioners incorporate some functional nutritional counseling along with traditional dietary recommendations which focus on the energetics of food. Though a raw, living food diet is avoided by many TCM practitioners, it is my belief that its anti-inflammatory nature and high concentration of phytonutrients make it a perfect remedy for the current prevalence of disease related to *Heat-Toxin* and *Excess*.

The second branch of TCM is herbal medicine. Chinese Herbal Medicine has the most extensive meteria medica of any system of herbal medicine in the world and is still widely practiced today. One of the strengths of Chinese Herbal Medicine is the practice of designing specific herbal formulas for individual patients. It was common practice until recently to send patients off with packages of dried herbs for them to spend hours preparing at home. The current gold standard in clinical practice is granulated formulas which allow the patient to get the potency of the "raw" formula in the convenience of a capsule.

Acupuncture is the third branch of TCM. This is the insertion of tiny, single-use needles in specific points throughout the surface of the body. Acupuncture increases blood flow, boosts immune activity and reduces inflammation. Acupuncture triggers the release of specific neurotransmitters and neurotropic factors which positively affect mental function and help resolve pain. It also stimulates electrical activity in the nerves and facia which is beneficial for Musculo-skeletal and neurological conditions.

The fourth branch of TCM is *qi qong* (pronounced "chi gung"), which can be broken down into two types: external and internal. Internal *qi gong*, the more common of the two, consists of specific movements. It is often slow and meditative; however, it provides tremendous benefits to the cardio-vascular system, the nervous system and cognitive function. External *qi gong* is much like reiki or what may be referred to as "energy healing." The body and its organs have magnetic or energetic fields which can be measured by modern technology. An individual can balance and expand these magnetic fields through intrinsic mental focus and positive emotional states like gratitude or unconditional love, or through practices like internal *qi gong*, meditation and yoga. External *qi gong* consists of the practitioner elevating his or her own energy field and then holding space for the patient often with the practitioner's hands on or above the patient's body.

The fifth branch of TCM is lifestyle counseling. This includes counseling the patient on stress management techniques, sleep hygiene and other daily practices focused on bringing the patient's health back into balance. Most TCM practitioners are trained to a small degree in psychological counseling, as the mind is viewed as not separate from the body, however serious mental health issues are referred to licensed mental healthcare professionals.

Traditional Chinese Medicine has an important principle which sets it apart from modern conventional medicine. Treat the individual, not just the disease. An individual patient may present with a disease diagnosis; however, everyone has his or her own unique constitution dictating how we approach the diagnosis. *Gu* syndrome often presents with an initial constitutional diagnosis of *spleen qi deficiency* which may include signs of a compromised gut microbiome according to Dr. Fruehauf. Other likely constitutional diagnoses may include *liver qi stagnation* if the patient has a high level of stress, and *lung qi deficiency* in the case of a weak immune system.

I met Jennifer at Hippocrates Wellness in 2022 when she was already well on her way back to a healthy life. I am always inspired when a patient can teach me something new about an illness they have endured or a holistic therapy I had not considered. Jennifer is someone who has taken a difficult situation head-on. She came to me with a chief complaint of neuropathy. I have successfully treated many types of neuropathies in my career. The type of neuropathy Jennifer presented has become more common recently, however. The presentation is nerve pain throughout the whole body. We see this not just with Lyme disease, but with an increasing number of post-COVID patients as well.

The treatment principles for Jennifer's treatment were: 1) Move the blood as pain can be diagnosed as *blood stasis* in TCM, and 2) Tonify the *wei qi* (support the immune system). The more common presentation of peripheral neuropathy responds well to certain types of acupuncture. Meridian therapy, which I use frequently, can often make pain, tingling or numbness disappear almost instantly. This approach is great when we can target specific locations. When the nerve pain is deep and throughout the body, it becomes a different animal altogether. Fibromyalgia pain can present more systemically and often falls into the *deficiency* pain category in my experience, as opposed to *blood stasis* which is an excess condition. Many fibromyalgia patients benefit from acupuncture as it not only boosts endorphins (our built-in morphine-like neurotransmitters) in the moment, but also causes the body to produce new endorphin receptors over cumulative treatments. This post-viral infection systemic neuropathy as I will call it, has elements of both excess and deficiency and can be more difficult to treat. Jennifer responded well to the acupuncture, and it seems to have played a valuable role in her journey back to wellness. The qi gong, however, was surprisingly impactful.

I have practiced *tai chi* and *qi gong* since 1996. I have a Masters and a Clinical Doctorate in Traditional Chinese Medicine. I have also been trained in *reiki*, craniosacral therapy, *Jin Shin Jyutsu* (acutouch therapy) among several other medical and therapeutic massage techniques. All this is to say that it is only in the past year or two that I have started to bring *qi gong* into the clinic. It is the willingness of people like Jennifer and the overwhelming response from the few patients that I have used this with in conjunction with acupuncture needles that has given me the inspiration to incorporate it more and more. Jennifer was able to go longer without pain when we did the external *qi gong* with acupuncture. It has been great to be a part of Jennifer's wellness team and I know that her experience will help inspire others to have faith and to act when faced with similar conditions.

1. An Ancient Solution for Modern Diseases: "Gu Syndrome" and Chronic Inflammatory Diseases with Autoimmune Complications (An Interview with Heiner Fruehauf). Retrieved from https://classicalchinesemedicine.org/heiner-fruehauf-gu-syndrome-chronic-inflammation-autoimmune/

2. Gu Syndrome, Lurking Pathogens, and Long Covid: An Old Take on a New Disease. Retrieved from https://www.ncbi.nlm.nih.gov/pmc/articles/PMC8594969/#ref8

Chapter 14

As a Physician

Nyree Abdool, DO

The heart of medicine, in my belief, is found within each technique that has been used in my practice for many years. The foundational views are correlated to the body's genetic makeup along with the physical symptoms that happen. This is what transforms into a variety of interactions within the cells, organs, and all the body systems. The skeletal frame of the body's mechanics is fused together to create an optimal learning experience for the physician and patient. The dynamics that I have encountered in treating various situations for each unique client provide a different effect from what is encountered over periods of time. Not everyone experiences the same manifestation of healing and transformation. There are many factors that can determine how the body is able to handle what goes into it. Our stress levels and family interactions interplay certain experiences on how the body reacts to various treatments.

I find it most beneficial in the majority of my practice to find the root cause of why the body has malfunctioned. Whether it be emotional or physical causes that bring symptoms of illnesses and diseases to rise, it is highly important that the main factor is exposed. In my opinion, this is what makes me so different from many other doctors in my field. I love taking the time with each patient to study their life, behaviors, and routines. It makes treating people much more realistic and it helps define my passion for healing even deeper.

When I began treating my patients for Lyme disease, harmful chemicals and toxins, bacteria, and other critical diseases, I focused a lot on the gut and developed a system to encourage the body to use its natural designed flora to do the work intended. This was the case in how I treated Jennifer when she first arrived at my practice. She had already received an immense amount of treatment, and it was imperative for me to take it more slowly than what she was used to. Sometimes physicians tend to go to the extreme when they know their patient has already been hit with the "big stuff". What I mean by this is, infusing stem cells, NAD, and other supportive mineral infusions all at once or in larger amounts to get a mass detoxification. There are times that it calls for us to slow it down, be patient, and help discover a new path of healing that has not been experienced before.

Jennifer came with considerable knowledge from all of her combined experiences of the past treatments she had received. I was floored by how well she had handled being ill for such a long time. I will say that she was about 85% well when she first entered my clinic. Typically, with patients like her, tolerance levels of strong infusions are pretty high. We developed a wellness plan to keep her from going backwards by doing ozone therapy, stem cells, NAD, and chelation. In addition, I provided Jennifer with much needed support that would cover her entire well-being.

What could I do for Jennifer that wasn't done before, was something that I took into deep perspective. This was a woman who had a surplus of experience and knowledge into the different realms of treatment and healing. She knew her body more than most physicians. So, the initial things were heightened, and added factors of the emotional aspects were vital in the initial phase of her coming to my clinic for assistance.

Let's start with ozone therapy. It is super-charged oxygen and instead of using O2, we use O3. With that extra molecule, it allows the body to intake and assimilate a more refined healing and rejuvenates the blood with more oxygen. The bacteria, mold, Lyme, and pathogens go through a process we refer to as a "kill". It wades off the foreign particles in the blood through excretion. It is really important when working with people that they are prepared to take the time needed to allow this work to be done. Treatment must be successful in the order of the gut, liver, lymphatic system, kidneys and more. Tonifying and opening up the cells allows the "dying off" of the toxins to release what has been weakening the immune system and clean up the bloodstream.

UV light therapy has different focal points; with ozone therapy it is effective for all viruses. The process exposes blood to UV rays to stimulate the immune system. UV light adds energy to the red blood cells. It breaks down your own cells like an auto vaccination. The cells then build an immune response that allows your body to fight against foreign substances and create more antibodies, which allows the body to properly build itself back. This is the natural way. Everyone has their own genetic information. It's amazing what the body can do on its own with the right method of treatment.

For heavy metal poisoning, a process of chelation, which has been around for a very long time, is done to bind to the metals that the body can't break down. When those metals are inside the body, they can be toxic and interfere with normal body functions. So, by adding a chelate agent, the metals can be removed. Some of the metals that we find in treatment come from chemicals, food, pathogens, parasites, belief systems, and genetics (lineage), that affect the gut and the immune system. The good and bad flora help to increase oxygenation and clear out the presence of plaque, especially with cardiovascular patients, and hyper-coagulate the system in Lyme patients.

Another hot topic of treatment used in Jennifer's case was the transfusion of NAD (nicotinamide adenine dinucleotide). NAD is the coenzyme form of niacin (vitamin B3) and plays a role in DNA repair. Its main concept is that as we age, there is damage when the mitochondria are depleted.

As the central repair system for the body, stem cells are intricate in the overall development of new cells. Jennifer had previous experience with receiving stem cell treatments prior to coming to see me. We started making different components and administering stem cells in different ways than intravenously. The performance of stem cells can rid the body of Lyme or mold. They have a high immunogenic response. When administering these cells there may be an outpouring of removal of toxins. Major effects may happen if these are not administered correctly when the body is not prepared, meaning that too many treatments too often cannot handle the elimination of the toxins because of the overload, so the liver cannot process the release. Glutathione, in this case, can go in and clean up to help support the liver, thus taking the toxic burden and helping the body shift focus to what's left specific to Lyme. The stem cells can cross the blood brain barrier.

According to research and my personal experience, the body should be neutral before any extensive treatment can occur. For many of my patients, including Jennifer, it has been vital to treat the human body as a delicate vessel so it can properly handle the rejuvenation process.

Chapter 15

As a Nurse

Julie H. Stansbury, BSN, RN

I am honored to be writing an excerpt for this book. I first met Jennifer in November of 2019 and was immediately greeted with a warm personality, zest for life and eagerness for health. I never would have known the battles she has faced just by looking at her. Our first interaction was at an IV Hydration Spa where I am employed as a Registered Nurse.

My passions include helping others become the healthiest version of themselves. Jennifer and I immediately connected and have built a growing relationship sharing our own knowledge about the benefits of Intravenous Vitamin Infusion therapy. Throughout Jennifer's Exosome Stem Cell infusion, she has been coming to see me to receive a specific regimen of vitamins about three times a week.

Jennifer usually receives a combination of B5, B6, B-Complex, B12, Vitamin C, L-Taurine, Zinc and Glutathione in 1,000 ml of lactated ringer IV solution. Each vitamin serves its own purpose in this infusion to aid cells to function at their optimal ability. B5, or dexpanthenol, is used to help reduce stress and anxiety as well as promote wound healing. Vitamin B6 or pyridoxine is essential for cognitive function and boosting the immune system. As I have learned from Jennifer, brain fog is a huge symptom associated with Lyme disease and is probably one of the most detrimental symptoms. Vitamin B12 or methylcobalamin helps to increase much needed energy and metabolism to continue on with your day. Vitamin C or ascorbic acid is essential for boosting the immune system and to promote wound healing. Lymphocytes, or white blood cells, uptake Vitamin C to help cells attack pathogens in the body. Along with Vitamin C, its counterpart Zinc helps to regulate immune function. L- Taurine is included in the IV infusion to assist in lowering the cortisol levels and to supplement energy production.

The final nutrient, Glutathione, provides the most specific benefit to Jennifer's health goal. Glutathione, also known as the Master Antioxidant, is a very popular supplement to aid the body in combating chronic illness. Glutathione is a molecule created by the liver to assist in detoxification processes. As we age, and are exposed to toxins, pollution and stress, our natural levels of glutathione decrease. Administering glutathione to the body gives the liver the extra fuel it needs to prepare the body to detox from harmful toxins and pathogens. In Jennifer's case, glutathione is used to help prepare her body to receive the stem cells by reducing inflammation and oxidative stress within the body.

It is essential to support your liver, kidneys and cells while recovering from a chronic illness by fueling with proper nutrition and supplementing with IV vitamins. I have seen a huge improvement in Jennifer's physical, mental and spiritual health in the short time since we have started working together. Jennifer's commitment to her health through perseverance is what has enabled her to be able to tell her story today.

Chapter 16

As a Nurse Practitioner

Shannon R. Weber, ARNP

I first met Mrs. Jennifer Brower at Hippocrates Wellness in 2022. She came to me for a consultation. She is not a big complainer and is the one, I later learned, who takes care of everyone else. She was suffering! She was desperate to feel better and regain her life. Her major complaints were brain fog, body aches, balance issues, neuropathy and intractable insomnia, among other things. During her consultation, I learned that she had a long history of Lyme disease and mold toxicity. I had no idea how much she had been through, how much she had tried to get better. I was still hopeful; encouraging her was imperative. Unfortunately, she was dealing with a regression of her dis-ease and health challenges and she was experiencing significant symptom progression. Subjectively, this was following a second bout of diagnosed COVID-19 infection.

When I met her, she appeared fairly healthy. She downplayed her suffering because of her beautiful spirit. She did have visible gait issues (poor balance when walking). She didn't remember much of what we spoke about, so there was quite a bit of repetition in discussing our plan. She had an implanted port in her chest, which was not her first port as I recall. We discussed a plan to treat her Lyme disease and its co-infections. She had been through so many different regimens prior to meeting me that she was extremely well versed on anything I explained to her. She could practically finish my sentences. The treatment regimen was initiated with compliance.

After a few days she came back to me complaining of "some uncomfortable symptoms" - an understatement. I was concerned that she was having a Herxheimer reaction from the toxins created by the killing off of bacteria, mold and possibly biofilm breakdown. She was immediately started on toxin binders, which were effective. Because of her positive attitude and minimal complaining, it was not apparent how sick she actually was. It wasn't until I stayed in touch with her and continued working with her that I realized how much she was dealing with. Her symptoms did improve, but she continued to struggle. We tried just about everything I could recommend. She literally did *everything* her other caring providers and I could offer her. She would travel to me and Hippocrates, and she continued with her local providers. She also continued with remote providers doing energy therapies that I learned about from her.

In my professional opinion, she is healthier today, but she has more healing to do. She prays and I have prayed for her healing. What I hope for her more than anything is that she receives the support she needs and deserves from her loved ones so that she can continue a positive, productive, healthy outlook on life. This is the only way she will continue in a positive direction. I will support her in any way I can. She is lovely and would help anyone. She deserves a reciprocal attitude from anyone and everyone she encounters.

Unfortunately, Jennifer's journey is not unique to her. I want her readers to understand that *suffering is not normal* and should not be considered acceptable. Just because we are aging does not mean we should be in a state of dis-ease, especially progressively. The contents of this book are applicable to every single human being. We all have struggles or at least know others who are struggling. To me, struggling = suffering. What is the point of living a life of suffering? Think quality, not quantity. My personal favorite quote is from Abraham Lincoln: "And in the end it's not the years in a life, it's the life in the years." Amen!

Please...do not stay in your lane...as a provider, patient, friend or family member, especially if you understand this. Share what you have discovered, discover what has been shared and continue to grow in understanding about how our bodies are designed to heal. Don't give up or give in. For quality of life's sake - yours and your loved one's - learn how to give back what has been stolen by stressful, traumatic and toxic events.

Chapter 17

As a Chiropractor

Dr. Nathan Riddle, DC, CCWP

My name is Dr Nathan Riddle and I am a chiropractor in Ponte Vedra Beach, Florida. I also have a clinic in Rochester NY and I have been in practice for 15 years. I have a love for traditional chiropractic adjusting but I also have a certification in the science of human wellness through the International Chiropractic Association. This certification has given me the confidence to communicate and teach individuals that they have an innate intelligence to achieve spectacular health by eating, moving, and thinking well, and that there are certain raw materials we require as a species to maintain balance (or what we term "homeostasis"). Over the past four years I have had special training in helping individuals naturally reduce neuropathy symptoms, and in many cases, patients have reported complete resolution of the issues over time. When patients come to us experiencing weakness, burning, pain, numbness, tingling, muscle weakness and balance problems, we know that the nerves are damaged, which can cause a number of problems, such as poor blood flow to the nerves, high levels of sugar in the blood, infections and an overload of toxins. There are over 100 different causes of nerve damage and neuropathy.

Jennifer reported to me in January 2023 with complaints of burning in her feet and a history of low back issues. She had tried multiple mainstream medical approaches with little to no success. Jennifer also said she was using and had used many different practitioners, herbs, lotions, potions, modalities, and magical wizardry to get relief. The bottom line was that Jennifer was not going to stop searching for help until she got better, so I was honored to be on the team to help her get back in balance.

Clinically it was discovered Jennifer had multiple subluxation complexes throughout her spine. Subluxation has two devastating effects: 1. When vertebrae are "gummed down" and not moving properly, it can cause arthritis and pain over time. 2. It creates poor nerve and blood flow throughout the body. The brain is fed by the gentle oscillations of a healthy spine. If spinal joints are subluxated, the brain is literally nutrient-deficient! As a result of Jennifer's poor alignment, she had poor posture and "knots" in her supporting spinal muscles. Another clinical finding was she had sensory deficits in her feet - a sign of neuropathy. According to the Toronto Clinical scoring system for Peripheral Neuropathy, she had 41% sensory loss in the left foot and 35% loss in her right. That meant she had moderate to severe nerve damage, and because neuropathy is a progressive degenerative disorder, it would only get worse over time if left uncorrected.

Jennifer has a tenacity to get better, and she was not going to let this take her life over, like we have seen with so many other people. Fortunately for her, she has some amazing resources and access to the best-of-the-best natural and holistic practitioners to help. The Lyme and mold toxicity and their effects would not destroy her quality of life and well-being.

We put together a plan she could use at home and in the clinic. My recommendations included decompression low back therapy, spinal adjustments, whole body vibration, home low-level infrared light therapy, Rebuilder therapeutic digital nerve stimulation, Supplementation to create alkalinity and boost Nitric Oxide production, topical cream with L-Arginine and Shockwave therapy. The shockwave therapy penetrates deep into the soft tissue, causing microtrauma, or a new inflammatory condition to the treated area. This "new injury" triggers the body's natural healing response once again. The energy emitted into the area also causes the cells in the soft tissue to release certain bio-chemicals that intensify the body's natural healing process. These bio-chemicals allow for the building of an array of new microscopic blood vessels in the soft tissue.

After four months, Jennifer's posture, spinal range of motion, muscle tonicity, and sensory loss all improved! It is a pleasure working with Ms. Brower and I look forward to continued improvements and maintenance.

Chapter 18

As a Personal Trainer

Colleen Clarson

A trainer is usually more than a trainer. We are often confidants, advisors, and trusted partners. For some lucky ones...friends. In my personal training relationship with Jennifer, it has been that but so much more.

Many trainers are approached by potential clients with the desire to "get in shape," or "lose weight," or "tone up." All of these are valid reasons to work with a trainer of course. I always believed anyone who was willing to commit the time and resources to working out was someone I wanted to use my resources to help.

Jennifer's story was different. In our relatively small town, most families with school-age children were bound to cross paths somewhere. Jennifer and I often worked together in the classroom, on fundraising efforts and representing the schools in our community. Jennifer had mentioned in casual conversations how much she enjoyed being active, working out and working in sports event marketing.

Both our families were active in our church. Our children went on mission trips together, served together at church services and were well-connected with all their church peers. During the time that our children were in middle and high school, there began to be talked-about concern for the Browers. There was much uncertainty, but subdued whispers were that *something* had happened. Was their house struck by lightning? Was Mrs. Brower very ill? Was their house consumed by mold and why did they have to move? Nobody seemed to have answers. It was just accepted that something was wrong. Jennifer and I lost touch for some time after that period of silence. She was not around much, and when she was, she didn't seem like herself.

In the meantime I became certified as a personal trainer and began training clients at the club where the Browers were members. One day as I was training a client, Jennifer's son Jennings went out of his way to seek me out in the gym. He thought his mom really needed to start working out again but that she probably needed a nudge. He asked if it would be OK if he gave her my contact information. Shortly thereafter, Jennifer called me.

In all my years of training, nobody had ever asked to meet me privately outside of the gym. I got an inkling that this would be something completely different from any of my previous client experiences. When we met, she looked like the same Jennifer I remembered. However, she sounded different. After a quick hug, she asked me if I was familiar with Lyme disease. She spoke about her terror with it and the subsequent horror of her family's suffering from a mold-infested home. She asked me to look at some websites with detailed information about how Lyme disease affects people and what they go through. Jennifer felt that she was fighting a war against her own body, and she wanted to get her health and fitness back.

The physical limitations that Jennifer had been experiencing stemmed from the medical challenges that affected her ability to work out like she used to. She urged me to not take it easy on her due to these issues, but to understand that some things may be more difficult to do than before. She asked me to look at a few websites, think about the challenges we might encounter, then just let her know if I would be willing to take on the challenge to work with her.

I was excited about the opportunity and considered it a great privilege to partner with her on her road to wellness. We started with an assessment of her current condition, identifying her goals, and creating a plan with timeline benchmarks. I told her if we couldn't laugh and have fun it likely wouldn't last for either of us. I became acutely aware of how much of her life she felt she could reclaim by a fitness routine, and I was highly motivated to help her achieve it. The old Jennifer laugh that I remembered came back! She raised her hand into a high-five and said, "Let's go!"

We began training together in 2016. Jennifer was very bothered by her loss of balance as well as the strength on her left side, particularly her left leg. We explored the full gamut of training modalities that would help her achieve her goals. When we first started, Jennifer was very wobbly in her balance and would often stumble or trip around the gym. I had to quickly get up to speed on what she could do that would be productive but challenging without putting her in any danger. Our goals were to make each workout focus on functionality and moving and working in ways that mirrored how we move throughout the activities of daily living. Outlined below were the key strengths and benefits goals:

*Increase overall fitness, strength, and endurance

*Improve strength on left side to align with right side strength

*Improve coordination of left side and especially left leg

*Improve core strength to assist with above goals

*Improve glute strength to assist with above goals

*HAVE FUN!

Mondays were for cardio and intervals with lighter weights. Wednesdays were for strength and power, and Friday included a combination of both. Every session included core work and functionality in all planes. A typical Monday might include jump squats, mountain climbers, modified burpees, TRX, quick dumbbell intervals and BOSU work for balance, core, and cardio. A typical Wednesday might include free weights and machines focused on all major muscle groups with special emphasis on legs (i.e., leg press, leg curl, walking weighted lunges, etc.). Sometimes we'd head outside and do a "bootcamp" workout utilizing resistance bands, kettlebells and light dumbbells, step-ups, pushups, dips, and other exercises utilizing the children's playground area on the sand. We also enjoyed putting our towels down on the sand for a full core workout.

After about a year and a half, Jennifer and I created a new method of training. Essentially it became a bootcamp which we did three to four days a week. The emphasis was on MOVING. The key element to most everyone's fitness and wellness is to keep moving, whatever that entails. I always told my clients the best form of working out for them was the one *that they would do*. While our focus remained on the earlier-set goals, we laughed more than ever and had more fun than ever. The time seemed to fly by.

We modified the workouts to implement resistance bands, medicine ball, free weights, and power walking. We started many workouts with a power walk and ended with core work and stretching on a mat. We had interval days, power & amp, strength and endurance days. We never ended a workout regretting that we made the effort to do it.

There were times that Jennifer simply didn't sleep well or felt crummy during the night. On those days I'd wake up to a text she sent me at 4am explaining that it had been a rough night and could we re-group for the following day. Those days were uncommon, but we have to give way to our bodies when we're simply not up to it.

A few months later we entered 'Phase 3'. We began a regimen of three to four times a week of briskly-paced power walks through the neighborhood, anywhere from 30 – 60 minutes each. We sometimes incorporated high intensity, faster-paced intervals into the walk to maximize cardiovascular benefits.

As time went on, I gave Jennifer a ten-pound weighted vest to wear to maximize her efforts and results while power walking. This enabled us to continue to build strength in Jennifer's leg, work on balance and move functionally as we do in our daily lives. We added in bodyweight strength training during the power walk by stopping at our favorite wood bridge. Jennifer would announce when we arrived at the bridge "C'mon nature, we're here, show us what you've got!" As if on cue, we would see a variety of wildlife which could include eagles, alligators, turtles, birds, and fish. We embraced our opportunities for fitness by making it a seamless part of our lives. I saw very noticeable improvement over the years in Jennifer's left leg strength and coordination, as well as overall and core strength. She continues to supplement our workouts with her own regular ocean and pool swims, a fabulous full-body workout.

Even during our nation's COVID-19 pandemic, we continued our workouts every day, maintaining social distancing as recommended. I look forward to helping her continue her progress to combat the diseases she is fighting.

Chapter 19

As a Caregiver

Ward Jones (1931-2022)

I had the honor of being a caregiver to Jennifer and wanted to share my overall insight. It was a great learning experience, as Jennifer told me it would be. Doing this for Jennifer was a privilege. Listening and experiencing this side of healing with Jennifer has helped both of us.

After dealing with Lyme and mold disease for 14 years, which as of this writing is cured, it was evident the process was draining for her. You have to bring back to life the body from the inside out. "You help the body – the body helps you, and the body heals itself." God allows us to heal our bodies if we listen to what our bodies are calling for: to live normal, happy, and loving lives!

I observed how intense and unique the healing plans were. She displayed a lot of courage and boldness. Some days, she would feel different emotions relating to her physical process. It was around the fourth day with her that I saw the effects of how she was recovering from the live stem cells. Stem cells are a vital aspect of healing and regeneration. These are the cells that enhance the good cells and rid the body of the bad cells. They are what lets the patient live in good health and happiness.

On day five, a booster treatment to power up the stem cells was given to Jennifer. It is nothing short of a miracle that the patient can *feel* the cleansing taking place and in the areas that the healing is needed. Patients also need positive thinking, which is a very important trait to have as a caregiver. Just being able to be with Jennifer, showing her support, love, faith, and hope, helped her to heal more quickly.

Having a greater knowledge and appreciation of what she is to me, has gone through, and the progress of these ongoing treatments, it is very clear that her healing is well-deserved. It has been an overwhelming honor and privilege to be the caregiver through this healing phase of Jennifer's life, as well as a learning experience that I will always cherish.

Part 3: Walking the Walk

There are so many people who inspire change and make a difference. I felt it would benefit my readers to learn the experiences of two particular women during my journey. Both Helena and Rahkia became forever friends of mine – some of the beauty that arose from the ashes of my illnesses.

Chapter 20

Sharing Strength

As a Friend and Advocate — Helena Bould

Having read up to this point in the book, you'll have already gleaned a tremendous amount of information as you search for your own solution to Lyme Disease, with or without additional health issues that are lowering your immune system. Hopefully, you've also had a chuckle or two at a number of the humorous stories.

We first met Jennifer when our youngest son Tom became a patient at a world-renowned integrative clinic in Florida, known for practicing alternative modalities alongside modern medicine.

As serious as things were at this clinic, laughter and supporting one another was a large element that significantly helped healing. Everyone fought their own paths to wind up there, but despite the severity of illness, patients bonded over telling their stories, and the caregivers present learned from one another. We all quickly became friends and advocates through the commonality of ailments.

People admitted to these specialty clinics are extremely sick, and in most cases have been given earlier misdiagnoses or even been told they aren't sick at all. As difficult as Lyme disease is, to then be told "it's all in your head," is gut-wrenching. Many patients had traveled all over the USA to other well-known clinics for answers; some had even traveled internationally only to return with nothing more than holes in their bank accounts. In many cases the treatment, or lack thereof, for Lyme can be determined by your insurance company, what state you are in, and CDC limitations imposed. Many such clinics don't deal at all with health insurance companies, leaving it up to the patient (or their advocate) to fight it out as the bills start rolling in.

One simple example of friends helping friends was the time Jen needed a ride to a not-so-local surgical center, an hour's drive away, for a procedure requiring some anesthesia. She thought she'd be okay to drive herself back! Not only did I offer to drive her there and back, but quite literally became her advocate in the surgical center (with her permission of course), so much so that the physician performing her procedure assumed we were sisters. We didn't correct him, and right there our bond was sealed.

On other separate occasions some patients and caregivers had insurance/billing questions, some needed a runner to a local health food store, or just a smoothie to be picked up from across the street. Whenever we advocates learned of or overheard that something was needed by our new friends, we endeavored to be there for them as much as we were there for our own. Many people at the clinic had no one with them for support. They were their own advocates, but having to be that when you are the patient, feeling desperately unwell and undergoing therapies, must be such a stress. My personal hope was that the gestures and help that I gave to others might alleviate some of that angst, stress and anxiety, allowing them to conserve their energy for healing. Often someone just needed an ear to listen to their frustrations and to have a kind word said. Support is crucial when you or a loved one deals with a chronic illness. As his mum, I'd naturally been Tom's advocate for the previous 2 years as we navigated his way through multiple fruitless specialist appointments.

Another of my favorite memories with Jen was when we'd become so close that we decided to share lodging while she and Tom were attending the clinic. It was prescribed that they both needed IV treatments during the evening hours. Since gravity is required for an IV line to function, the challenge was to find "hooks" high enough in the sitting room to suspend the IV bags from! What a sight it was to see their IV bags dangling from light fittings, chandeliers or picture hooks!

I'd like to share Tom's story with you.

Some of what I have to share is different from Jen's experiences since initial symptoms can differ from one patient to the next (yes, Lyme does mimic over 300 autoimmune diseases), but over time certain symptoms associated with Lyme Disease generally become universal among patients.

In 2015, I first recognized a shift in our 17-year-old son Tom's overall demeanor. He wasn't concentrating like he used to – homework that he typically breezed through in one hour became a monstrous task that took over 3 hours to complete. He was experiencing the classic signs of brain fog, but didn't think he was sick.

I'd recently recovered from my own battle with Lyme; so I was only too familiar with it, and despite my suspicion, our doctor couldn't confirm that Tom had Lyme since his blood work didn't quite fit the "positive" interpretation according to CDC criteria.

Tom then started to grumble about aches and pains in his joints and uncharacteristically became very angry at minor situations that would never have fazed him before. He'd snap and snarl at the slightest of comments and then in the next breath apologize with tears welling up in his eyes as he simply didn't know, and couldn't explain, where that anger and raw emotion had come from. "Lyme Rage" is real.

He experienced overwhelming lethargy and chronic fatigue. His primary care physician believed the aches and pains were typical for someone his age associated with the rigors of playing academy-level soccer and weight training. By the spring semester of 2016 Tom totally lacked the passion for the sport he so loved, and soon confessed he was feeling desperately unwell and needed help.

Tom's greatest complaint was his jaw. He experienced unbelievable headaches and his bite had completely changed - he recognized himself that he couldn't even chew properly! The first specialist we saw was his dentist who informed us that his bottom jaw had indeed shifted approximately 3/4 of a tooth towards his right ear!

Over the next year, the quest to find any plausible reasoning and potential solution sent us to an orthodontist, an ENT specialist, a sleep therapist, a sacro-cranial specialist, a TMJ expert, chiropractors, and an oral surgeon. Each specialist was equally flummoxed.

Administrators at Tom's school wondered if the headaches could possibly be concussion-related to soccer and repeated "heading" of the ball during training and games. Long story short, Tom underwent various treatments and therapies for "post-concussion syndrome." This was one of many rabbit holes we went down.

Regardless, we decided to assume it was Lyme and Tom decided to get strict on the Lyme diet. It initially helped but wasn't a cure.

Eventually, we found a specialist where Tom tested positive for Lyme according to the results from the iSpot Lyme test, which is not approved by the CDC in the USA but is used in Germany and Australia.

Tom's appointment with the Lyme specialist was a breath of fresh air. He stated that had he been able to see Tom one year earlier he would have started him immediately on treatment for Lyme based on his symptomatology and the Western Blot alone. It's a real dilemma faced by physicians – Do you play Russian roulette with a person's life by deciding not to treat them just because they don't fit the CDC criteria? Do you allow them to become chronic just because they don't fit a mold? According to the CDC, chronic Lyme still does not exist! Maddening!

Tom's treatment for Lyme started exactly 12 months after I'd first seen the warning signs. We revisited some of the specialists he'd seen: Pre-diagnosis, both the TMJ specialist and the oral surgeon had said there was nothing wrong with his MRI, it was completely unremarkable, and they were at a loss as to how or why his lower jaw had shifted, even though they could see that it clearly had. When we later told them we had "new news to share," both specialists had "Aha!" reactions, and both acknowledged, "Yes, Lyme can do this." *They had not thought outside their own specialist boxes* until we gave them the news.

Tom continued to experience pain around his head, neck, jaw, shoulder, and lower back. Regular massage therapy alleviated some pressure. The chiropractor discovered through X-ray that his spine from the shoulders to the base of his skull, the cervical vertebrae, was off-axis and leaning to the right. A rigorous schedule of physical therapy was added to the calendar that included dry needling among the various techniques used to alleviate his oral-facial pain and jaw disorder. This cycle continued for over a year, including a PICC line for his IV antibiotics with no significant improvement. In fact, Tom didn't get worse, but he wasn't getting any better.

Our quest for help and to get Tom healthy led us to the specialty clinic in Florida, where his blood work showed *two* different strains of Lyme bacteria. He had both the predominant American Lyme, Borrelia burgdorferi, *and* the predominant European Lyme, Borrelia afzelii.

Shockingly, in addition to his Lyme diagnosis, we found he was riddled with industrial toxicants (petrochemicals) and mold toxins. Tom's results also showed a significant amount of biofilm in his blood, which included some parasites. He also had a very weakened gut - "leaky gut" - and suppressed hormone levels.

In Tom's early years, he'd played soccer on a contaminated grass field which had been New Jersey's largest polymer factory. This is quite possibly where Tom was exposed to the petrochemicals.

To name one, acrylamide was one of the petrochemicals that presented itself in his blood work at limits well beyond acceptable. Where had that come from? These petrochemicals are used in many industrial processes such as plastics, food packaging and dyes. It is also found in potato chips and french fries. The doctor at our clinic had even treated the daughter of Europe's largest private producer of acrylamide. Back then in Europe, acrylamide was used by certain fast food restaurants to stiffen their french fries!

Testing had also revealed that Tom's gut absorbency of essential amino acids was so poor that it apparently "compared to a 90-year-old in a nursing home." He was undernourished as his body wasn't absorbing anything.

We wondered how and when Tom was exposed to mold. During a home renovation project, we realized that for the first five years of living in our home, we'd unquestionably had a leaky window in the basement where our young boys spent most of their time playing. When we moved into the house, Tom was only 2.5 years old, an age at which an immature liver can't readily process toxins. And, through genetic testing, we learned that Tom has the HLA-DR gene, meaning he does not process mold toxins readily. His poor body had accumulated toxins all of his life, so when he did eventually get bitten by a tick (or by an infected spider), his immune system simply couldn't cope.

One of the mold toxins that came out of Tom's biofilm was Ochratoxin A. An acceptable level is 1.2. Tom's level was 13.8!

"Ochratoxin A (OTA) is a nephrotoxic, immunotoxic, and carcinogenic mycotoxin. This chemical is produced by molds in the Aspergillus and Penicillium families. Exposure is primarily through contaminated foods such as cereals, grape juices, dairy, spices, wine, dried vine fruit, and coffee. Exposure to OTA can also come from inhalation exposure in water-damaged buildings. OTA can lead to kidney disease and adverse neurological effects. Studies have shown that OTA can cause significant oxidative damage to multiple brain regions and the kidneys. Dopamine levels in the brain of mice have been shown to be decreased after exposure to OTA" - The Great Plains Laboratory.

Mold toxins can damage your cartilage and tendons and erode the myelin sheaths on your nerves. Was this the cause of all his aches and pains?

By using detoxification protocols, Tom went through a cycle of "kills". This took its toll on his already exhausted body. He would wake up each morning feeling like someone had taken a sledgehammer and whacked him over the head, hard. He hardly had any energy.

Through continued rounds of detoxification and immune-boosting protocols, the clinic cleaned many of these toxins out of him and thereby improved not only his leaky gut, but reversed kidney, thyroid, and male hormone imbalances.

After a month of detoxing molds and petrochemicals, he was prescribed a 2-week course of IV antibiotics for the Lyme. His blood results came back some time later showing that treatment had worked and the Lyme, plus his co-infections were under control. Additional specialist blood work gave us high-resolution images of Tom's red blood cells looking much healthier.

We were advised that after these intensive treatments, many patients are so sensitive to their environment they often experience reactions to a contaminated environment within minutes of entry. Tom was warned that this sensitivity could give him the skill set of a sniffer dog! Within his first week of being at home, this did happen. He walked into a friend's basement, one that he had practically lived in with his buddies, and experienced an immediate reaction. His neck stiffened up, he developed ringing in the ears and a headache all within minutes of walking into that room. Tom made his polite excuses and came home to a house that we'd made as safe as we possibly could.

It's certainly been a journey. A five-year journey. The lessons we've learned are:

- If the doctors can't provide answers to the questions you have, keep going.

- Find an advocate who can support you and if not, recognize that you may have to be your own.

- For Tom, without the support of family, friends, acquaintances, doctors, nurses, and prayers said, healing wouldn't have been possible. One can never truly measure the importance that "support" provides. But know this: support is vital.

You will get there - Jen & Tom are testaments to that.

Chapter 21

Experiencing the Mission

As I was praying about writing a book, I knew I needed the help of someone who understood patient interaction and scientific testing, and Rahkia came to my mind. She had worked for a doctor, understood test results and run interference with patients.

Rahkia Millerd, MS — As an Advocate for Jennifer's Health and her Book

It was a bright and sunny day on a family vacation near home. A perfect setting to think about life while relaxing underneath the cabana. Then my phone rang. What a thrill and unexpected surprise to hear Jennifer's voice on the other end of the phone! It had been a few months since we last connected, but our hearts were always tied together since meeting at the clinic where she had been a patient.

Because of my recent transition from a former employer, I had available time to collaborate on this journey with Jennifer to tell her story. A word that sparked our flames was "global". Along with her experience of business and travel, my calling to write books and poetry, and my added devotion to the mental health field, we were preparing to embark on a course from which we would never look back. I admit that this process has not been a breeze, but with persistence and courage, we sought to journal our experiences together and share Jennifer's trials while going through various treatments. Every moment and chance to write, we did just that! Sitting in the sauna, walking along the beach, at dinner, lying down when we both had no energy, facetime calls, at the airports, by the pool, in our offices, and especially while Jennifer was receiving treatment, we kept our minds open to jot as much down as we could.

So here we are now at the end of this book. It is our strong desire that you have gained a new outlook on your personal life, the well-being of others, and plan to jump-start your health with a renewed mind and confidence. There are many books that you could have read and I thank you for choosing this one. Now, let me begin with a few things that this dream of writing Jennifer's story has created, and also what I have experienced.

Knowing Jennifer has been the most amazing experience and relationship discovered in my lifetime. The path she has taken to gain every ounce of power, healing, motivation and force is phenomenal and inspiring. Her life's story has changed me profoundly. The devoted passion she exudes in everything she does has been remarkable. Her heart fully cares for those who are trying to find answers, leading them to healing from the inside and outside, and finding who they are within themselves.

As my relationship with Jennifer has strengthened, the next level of ventures has opened widely to sharing our visions with many people we come into contact with. It ministers to our hearts as we speak on life experiences, trials and errors, and the successes we have achieved. It is most interesting when two people from vastly different walks of life meet but have so much in common. If you ever want to get to know how it feels to walk in someone else's shoes, just sit with them and talk about things that mean the most to them. Healing is sure to satisfy the soul and relieve the most deprived and wounded. This is the subject that sealed our future and that would bring us to the point to write about all we have been through, and reach your hearts.

It is also my great pleasure to share my points of view of the in-person experiences that I have witnessed with Jennifer undergoing treatment and using unique modalities to assist her. All these efforts were made to achieve goals of healing inwardly and outwardly. Before I explore these snippets with you, I would like to tell you how we met. You just never know whom you will meet, so it pays off to be kind to all you encounter, and most of all, a smile and a hug goes a million miles!

In July of 2017, I had the opportunity to work for a renowned physician in Oldsmar, Florida who specializes in integrative medicine treating patients from all over the world. With diagnoses of Lyme disease, mold toxicity, environmental chemicals and parasitic diseases, the patients desperately needed healing. People were searching for answers, and everywhere they turned, doors were closed. Entering this clinic was a breakthrough moment that many felt was the last resort. This breaking moment is what healing is all about. This is where I met Jennifer. Her strength drew me, and my life has never been the same.

The presence that Jennifer carried as she walked into the clinic daily was uplifting, charismatic, powerful, and conquering. She had a willingness to face everything that was invading her body. Her determination and strength are what brought change from the inside out. Yet, she also made sure that others had their chances to get on the right path to their own healing. I have witnessed Jennifer pouring her heart out through time, commitment, pursuit of results and satisfaction for others. Just like she fights for her family, she did the same for everyone she encountered. As I would sit and talk with Jennifer, her countenance would always intrigue me. She has so much love in her heart that caring for others is natural. Her life was busy, yet she still made time for everyone.

These are some of the experiences I have been able to witness throughout Jennifer's healing journey. They have all presented eye-opening changes in my own life. I do feel that it is important to take the time to be with your loved ones while they are going through therapies and treatments as much as possible. Until you walk in their shoes, it may be difficult to see how much is required to have a balanced and normal life. Having family or close friends near plays a vital role in the healing process. Empathy and compassion are powerful mind tools to display when providing support to a sick loved one.

The treatments Jennifer received were highly sensitive in nature and administered with caution. During one particular treatment session, she received a buccal intermuscular shot of stem cells. Dr. Nyree, a phenomenal holistic medical physician, used special gloves to remove the FDA-registered stem cells from the box. She held the frozen vials in her hand to defrost them. It was to set the intention of healing within through the transmission of the stem cells. She then placed them in Jennifer's possession, and she opened the bag containing the vials.

The anticipation, expectation, confidence, and prayer that went forth before administering the stem cells was vital. The process was delicate and precise. Every second was intentional in this life-changing moment of continued healing. Calmness, silence, and a flow of embrace, the therapeutic process was setting intentions on the highest level of healing and success. The atmosphere was charged with energy and salience to remove any foreign and spiritual toxins that would infiltrate or block the manifestation of the cells from accomplishing the body's goals. After this moment, the doctor prepared the setup with expertise and brilliance. The difference between this and previous experiences was the careful planning. I was amazed by how the environment changed the moment the box of cells was opened. It was as if the cells were destined for Jennifer.

It was then time for the stem cells to settle and do their work. Dr. Nyree smoothed Gentle Baby essential oil onto Jennifer's arms and the healing began. No interruptions during this moment. Every ounce of focus was set on the entry and follow-through of the stems doing their part inside the human body. An IV bag of glutathione was given after the stem cells injection. Jennifer said she felt that things were moving in and around her muscles. She felt tense and tight (which is to be expected after receiving an injection in that area), her senses were becoming heightened, following the rush of a cooling sensation in her brain, and a calm flow over her entire body.

A blood analysis was completed before and after the stem cells were given. I observed on the imaging screen her red blood cells and their irregular forms. The results were amazing after the stem cells. Her red blood cells took a complete turn and appeared healthier than before! The heavy metal toxins were not visible, and the uric acid was removed from her bloodstream.

When the next treatment session began, tension began releasing from the upper region of Jennifer's body. She prepared by stretching to elongate her physique and to aid the process of a refining grounding moment. Dr. Nyree conducted a deep meditation that penetrated the room, along with the sound of sweet waves and a delicate prayer over the stem cells. No extra movement or hindrance would intrude that space. And again, I was amazed by the poise of the doctor while preparing for this delicate treatment. Few doctors are willing to take as much time to ensure their patients are comfortable and peacefully prepared for their treatments. They tend to leave that to the nursing staff.

Jennifer has opened my mind to many unique techniques that I had not heard of or even contemplated trying on my own. Magnetic therapy, or biomagnetism, is used to treat many conditions and different types of pain and insomnia. Though research is still being conducted of its overall uses and benefits, biomagnetism can be used in conjunction with other treatments like acupuncture. While observing Jennifer undergoing a magnetic therapy session, I took a few notes with the help of therapist Ralph Sorreno. He learned this technique in Mexico City and has developed his expertise through training and hands-on experiences.

Biomagnetism is used in conjunction with kinesiology, whereby the body is checked for imbalances, impurities, fungi, viruses, and bacteria. Magnetic therapy is the use of negative and positive pressure that have the potential to change its polarization. Since magnetic therapy is not a one-time fix, it is recommended that a minimum of four sessions be undertaken to focus on the debilitating challenges that are presented, for example, cancers and fibromyalgia. Glandular and emotional issues are also areas of focus for this therapy. The therapist shared that between 8 and 22 minutes, the body is able to rebalance for the magnetic fields to clear. The fingers and feet tend to get cold during these sessions.

The process started with deep breathing and grounding. As the therapist set up, magnets were placed on the front and back of the knees, two on both sides of the upper collar bone of the chest, the upper right quadrant and under the wrists. Eye patches were positioned while Jennifer was reclining. The therapist held and bounced the feet at the heels. He was guided through the phone (which can help alter changes) while asking Jennifer specific questions. If the right foot moved upward, that indicated there was an imbalance in that area, and he knew what to treat from there. Other therapists are known to use the tens unit. For this particular session, the therapist began working on the areas of Jennifer's gallbladder and food intake. It was noted that her blood sugar was elevated, and indications of stress were revealed. Her body was less acidic than prior sessions, as it lined up with blood analysis completed on the same day as the stem cell treatment. Once again, she was advised to eliminate dairy (which she wasn't consuming anyway). There were also indicators that Lyme was lying dormant, though no spirochetes were shown in the first blood draw for the blood analysis. There was pain in her legs, right knee, and the arches of her feet. This let the therapist know what he needed to work on as well. Her nervous system, gallbladder, and the intestines were moving more slowly. The lungs appeared clear, and sleep would be an issue to work on.

Improving the central nervous system (CNS) is essential for Jennifer as it has been immensely better, but due to COVID-19, the imbalance of her CNS enhanced her sensitivities, especially when she had any type of infection or inflammation.

During that moment, Jennifer felt that things were still balancing in her brain. When the magnets were placed, her body felt relieved and calmer. After everything was over, Jennifer had a glow that expressed happiness, relief and hope. Her body balanced very well. Results indicated that Jennifer tolerated the stem cells in a perfect and resolute way.

During a different session Jennifer was having electrical shooting pains from her abdomen to her heart. Though these significations may be painful, the magnets can take some time to do their proper work. The summer of 2021 was the first time we heard mention of Jennifer's liver function. She was advised to eliminate celery juice for four days, then she could gradually reintroduce it, starting with eight ounces once a day, then gradually increasing to twice a day, then after a week, increasing to ten ounces twice a day, and so on. The therapist was unaware of the wound site and he happened to place the magnets on the actual wound area. That was right on point! There were intense sensations felt from that area, which implied that the magnets were doing their job to help alleviate the pain she had been experiencing.

During a recent stay at the Hippocrates Wellness with Jennifer, my personal approach to wellness was in for a big transformation. From eating raw organic vegetables to wheatgrass and green juice twice daily, our careful consumption of food was sure to improve our food habits at home. Lifestyle improvement was the biggest component to securing a positive mindset of what goes into our bodies. We were taught many things, from properly preparing and growing organic sprouts (the main component of daily meals) to which foods cause disease and how to improve our mental capacity (meditation, healing groups, exercise, etc.). And we heard various lectures based on attainable and realistic information. No salt or sugar was found in our meals, and the substitutions were all organic. Everything prepared for us daily had a purpose for our internal and external bodies. The staff was highly educated. The property was serene and therapeutic, and great relationships were formed. Oh, before I forget, the mineral, salt, and cold plunge pools were a must to partake in! The best, healthiest retreat I must say.

The immunity protocol that Jennifer was enrolled in included plans to help boost her immune system, rid toxins through proper means of detox - juicing, sauna, lymphatic tissue drainage, IV compilations (used on patients with Lyme disease, cancer, and other major illnesses), the use of the hyperbaric chamber, massage and much more. Throughout her 3-week stay, her schedule was extremely busy. A full night's rest was something Jennifer had continued to struggle with over the past decade and going through this transformation provided a better routine and pattern to rest. Pain was also addressed at Hippocrates. The severity and longevity of Jennifer's back pain, as well as sciatica, became minimal at certain points. Regaining her physical mobility to complete lengthier exercises and workout routines began as well.

Jennifer described this transformation period as being at Disney World, on the moving sidewalk of Space Mountain, looking into Future Land. It gave a feeling that opened her eyes to a new life - a moving pathway that takes you through a course to get the grand result desired. The many therapies that were involved with the overall immunity were outstanding. Every aspect of life was channeled through this place. The core advice was to stand strong and remain consistent.

With amazement from the firsthand experiences of watching Jennifer heal, I have learned that the body is able to heal from within. There are times the body needs a jumpstart. Using different physical, spiritual, and emotional techniques and modalities is effective in healing. Continual healing renews your faith and unleashes the potential for a stronger and healthier self.

Courage comes in and the fear starts to dissipate when you take baby steps to get to the healing process. You will be able to think clearly which will in turn bring great success. We can always observe what someone else is going through or try to evaluate life from a different perspective.

On the basis of treatment, we are too used to "textbook" methods, rather than tackling the heart of the problem. Take a step into the eastern and western methods to explore for your health. Functional methods can be a great way to get the body to function better than you can imagine. What will it take to go beyond your own thinking and reach beyond all limits? You can do it!

Afterword

How to prepare yourself and your family

My advice to spouses and family members of those diagnosed with Lyme disease: Be present (not just in the *initial* meeting with the doctor - there will be *many*), hold your loved one's hand, and make it your business to understand the process of the treatment. Say to your loved one, "You are safe; I am with you." All of these things will help smooth the healing and recovery.

1. Doctors, scientists, and clinics that specialize in treating Lyme disease often do not take insurance and expect payment at the time of treatment. I have watched other patients make huge financial (homes, savings, all worldly belongings) and personal (family, marriages, and friendships) sacrifices to fully recover from Lyme disease. The good news is that now some blood and urine tests are covered by insurance and that Lyme is now test-worthy.

2. Different treatments work for different people who have Lyme disease. It is an auto-immune disease that will manifest itself distinctly in different people. You will have your own personal journey that will not look exactly like mine.

3. Stages: diagnosis of the disease, relief of symptoms, treatment of the disease, and healing and repairing the effects of the disease. All stages need to be addressed, and specifically-trained doctors and scientists may be better at dealing with each stage.

4. When a person's leg is broken, you see them on crutches and in a cast, so you know what the presenting issue is. Such is not the case with Lyme disease or mold toxicity. It is almost 100% internal. Therefore, you will have to communicate how you are feeling to your loved ones and educate them about the diseases.

5. Beware of those who would take advantage of the fact that you're sick and try to persuade you to try their proposed "solution." They know you're vulnerable, perhaps even desperate, and will try to capitalize on that. Use discernment.

6. Build your own healing team, be it lay or medical professionals.

7. Hang on to the people who don't ditch you during a crisis!

> Many of the advanced treatments that helped Jennifer recover carry a hefty price tag. Remember, the core of healing is not costly. First, develop a positive mindset. Second, eat clean and nourishing organic plant food. Third, use water – hot and cold therapy in showers, baths, saunas, steam baths, etc. Fourth, magnets that are inexpensive can be employed on painful areas of the body and head. Fifth, and most important, your commitment to self-heal is what truly makes it happen.
>
> Brian Clement, PhD, LN.

I pray that the story of my journey has been helpful and insightful for you. Silent Killers has become more than a book. It's a community, and members of communities support one another. It is my sincere hope that you know you are not alone. I invite you to join my community by going to www.JenniferCBrower.com.

Acknowledgements

When I fell face down, my next-door neighbor Suzanne Franco ensured my family was taken care of. She took my kids to school and practices and ran any extra errands needed for their daily activities. Suzanne and her wonderful husband Bob's lasting friendship and enduring encouragement mean the world to my family.

Longtime friends Lisa and John Baccich have demonstrated continued love and support, even putting a roof over our heads as I finished writing this book.

Dr. Nyree Abdool found ways to provide the best healing mechanisms uniquely suitable for me. Her expertise is truly one-of-a-kind.

My dear friend, Helena Bould, who contributed to this book, knelt beside me during treatments with her son, and taught me more healthful ways of eating. Her passion for nutrition and healing is beyond imagination.

To all of the scientists, doctors, nurses, aides, techs, and medical professionals who contributed words of knowledge and expertise and assisted me by diving into this book and finding ways to bring healing to others, you will never be forgotten.

Dr. Maggie Gama is an absolute rockstar as a doctor, ongoing supporter and never-ending friend.

My ghost writer, Rahkia, helped me put this book together, stood by my dreams and visions, and believed in everything I sought to do. I am grateful for her love, devotion, friendship, partnership, and for being so real in my life.

ACKNOWLEDGEMENTS

The writing of this book began nearly three years ago, but the greatest blessing was the time the incredible, hard-working team came together as friends in the final months. We traveled from multiple cities and states to physically sit together for a week, engaging each other's strengths, brainstorming and bringing this book project to fruition:

- Melinda McManus, my editor

- Brittani Feinberg, my gatekeeper, website designer, negotiator, marketer, basically my "everything" manager

- Natalia Maldonado, my Mindset and Empowerment Coach

- Shannon Weber, my IV Specialist

My spiritual go-tos throughout my health-seeking journey were vital to my healing. Dr. Mercy D. Jones, my angel sent from heaven, who played an integral part in raising me *and* my children, was with me day in and day out while I was sick, stopping by before and after work. The Reverend Rick Westberry, the Reverend Sue Carmichael and my bible study group all were endlessly supportive of me, lifting me up and buoying my faith so that I had the strength to face each day.

Recommended Reading List

Medical Medium Collection by Anthony William

Self-Healing Diet by Dr. Brian Clement and Dr. Anna Maria Clement

Health Beauty by Dr. Samuel Epstein and Randall Fitzgerald

LifeForce by Dr. Brian Clement

Healing Our Autistic Children by Dr. Julie Buckley

Supplements Exposed by Dr. Brian Clement

Breast Cancer: Start Here: Everything You Need to Know About Integrative Health for the Newly Diagnosed by Dr. Julie Buckley

The Emotion Code by Dr. Bradley Nelson

References

Centers for Disease Control and Prevention. (2020). Basic Facts about Mold and Dampness. *National Center for Environmental Health.* Retrieved from https://www.cdc.gov/mold/faqs.htm

Centers for Disease Control and Prevention. (2019). Bartonella Infection (Cat Scratch Disease, Trench Fever, and Carrion's Disease). *National Center for Emerging and Zoonotic Infectious Diseases and Division of Vector-Borne Diseases.* Retrieved from https://www.cdc.gov/bartonella/clinicians/index.html

Centers for Disease Control and Prevention. (2019). Ehrlichiosis; Signs and Symptoms. *National Center for Emerging and Zoonotic Infectious Diseases and Division of Vector- Borne Diseases.* Retrieved from https://www.cdc.gov/ehrlichiosis/symptoms/index.html

Ellis, R. R. (2021). What is magnetic field therapy? *WebMD.* Retrieved from https://www.webmd.com/pain-management/magnetic-field-therapy-overview

Elvis, A. M., & Ekta, J. S. (2011). Ozone therapy: A clinical review. *Journal of natural science, biology, and medicine, 2*(1), 66–70. https://doi.org/10.4103/0976-9668.82319

Florida Times-Union. (2011). Ask UNF: Lyme disease in Florida – what you need to know. *Jacksonville.com/The Florida Times-Union.* Retrieved from: https://www.jacksonville.com/story/news/local/2011/06/09/ask-unf-lyme-disease-florida-what-you-need-know/15900862007/

Holze, C. (2016). Brain Nutrients for Chronic Lyme Disease. *Holze Wellness Center*. Retrieved from https://www.holzewellness.com/brain-nutrients-chronic-lyme-disease/

Marra, S. L. (2022). Glutamate Excitotoxicity. *EcoMedica*. Retrieved from https://drsusanmarra.com/2022/01/glutamate-excitotoxicity/.

Shapiro E. D. (2014). Borrelia burgdorferi (Lyme disease). *Pediatrics in review*, *35*(12), 500–509. Retrieved from https://doi.org/10.1542/pir.35-12-500

Wolfson, J. (2019). How Mold Can Cause Atrial Fibrillation. *TDW/TheDrsWolfson*. Retrieved from https://thedrswolfson.com/how-mold-can-cause-atrial-fibrillation/

Extra Resources:

Clausen, R. (n.d.). Infrared Sauna Therapy—New Hope for the Rising Number of Lyme Disease Cases. *Alternative Medicine News*. Retrieved from https://olli.gmu.edu/docstore/800docs/1401-807-How%20to%20Look%20and%20Feel%20Younger/Lyme%20Disease%20Alt%20Med%201110_Lyme.pdf

Nourished Blessings. (n.d.). Looking at Glutamate in Underlying Infections & Immune Dysfunction: Pans, Pandas, Ae, Lyme, etc.). Nourished Blessings. Retrieved from https://nourishedblessings.com/immune-function-underlying-infections-pans-pandas-lyme-etc/

Shalat, S. (2017). Does playing on artificial turf pose a health risk for your child? *The Washington Post*. Retrieved from https://www.washingtonpost.com/national/health-science/does-playing-on-artificial-turf-pose-a-health-risk-for-your-

child/2017/03/17/0c61b7b4-0380-11e7-ad5b-
d22680e18d10_story.html?utm_term=.012374df0efb

Tim. (2023). Clean, Remediate, Protect: How to DIY: Take home
health into your own hands. *Superstratum.* Retrieved from
https://superstratum.co/2023/07/07/clean-remediate-protect-
instructions/

U.S. Food and Drug Administration (updated 2022).Survey Data on
Acrylamide in Food. *FDA.* Retrieved from
https://www.fda.gov/Food/FoodborneIllnessContaminants/ChemicalC
ontaminants/ucm053549.htm

WebMD Editorial Contributors. (2022). High Glutamate Foods.
WebMD. Retrieved from https://www.webmd.com/diet/high-
glutamate-foods#3

WebMD Editorial Contributors. (2021). Health Benefits of Infrared
Saunas. *WebMD.* Retrieved from
https://www.webmd.com/balance/health-benefits-of-infrared-saunas

Scan the below QR code or go to www.silentkillersbook.com/resources

- To view any of this book's images in color and for further
  descriptions

- For websites of various health providers and book contributors

- For Jennifer's Helpful Health Hacks

To book Jennifer C. Brower for your next conference or in-house event, please contact:

Brittani Feinberg
Silent Killers Project Manager & Marketing Director
Silent Killers, LLC
250 A1A, Suite 100
Ponte Vedra Beach, FL 32082

Mobile: 904-944-2273
E-mail: Management@jennifercbrower.com
Website: www.jennifercbrower.com

Rahkia Millerd, M.S., Ghost Writer

Born and raised in Florida, Rahkia finds her passion and strength in mental health and writing. While married and raising 4 children, she reached one of her educational and career destinations in the field of psychology. She has also devoted much effort to the community through sharing her art as an author. Rahkia uses her writing gift to help those in need through their personal journey of healing. She is devoted to youth and adults who have experienced trauma and abuse, career conflict, depression and anxiety. Rahkia continues to encourage others with hope and purpose.

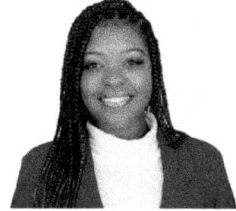

Brian Clement, Ph.D, L.N., Contributor

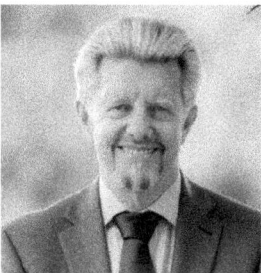

Brian is the Director of the internationally renowned Hippocrates Wellness, located in West Palm Beach, Florida. It's the world's leading center for working with affliction and reversing premature aging, and is frequented by the likes of Sir Anthony Hopkins, Elliot Page, Mick Fleetwood and Elle Macpherson. **For over 50 years**, Brian's limitless love and passion to mentor and guide hundreds of thousands of lives into a semblance of balance and well-being have led to countless hours of practical and clinical experience, positioning him as one of the world's leading progressive thinkers and teachers.